Breaking Free
of Managed Care

THE CLINICIAN'S TOOLBOX™
A Guilford Series

Edward L. Zuckerman, Series Editor

CLINICIAN'S THESAURUS, 4th Edition
The Guidebook for Writing Psychological Reports
Edward L. Zuckerman

CLINICIAN'S THESAURUS
Electronic Edition, Version 4.0
Edward L. Zuckerman

BREAKING FREE OF MANAGED CARE
A Step-by-Step Guide to Regaining Control
of Your Practice
Dana C. Ackley

Forthcoming

THE PAPER OFFICE, 2nd Edition
Forms, Guidelines, and Resources
Edward L. Zuckerman

BREAKING FREE OF MANAGED CARE

A Step-by-Step Guide to Regaining Control of Your Practice

Dana C. Ackley

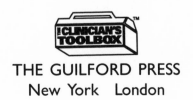

THE GUILFORD PRESS
New York   London

©1997 The Guilford Press
A Division of Guilford Publications
72 Spring Street, New York, NY 10012

Printed in the United States of America

This book is printed on acid-free paper.

Last digit is print number: 9   8   7   6   5   4   3   2

Library of Congress Cataloging-in-Publication Data
Ackley, Dana C.
    Breaking free of managed care : a step-by-step guide to
regaining control of your practice / by Dana C. Ackley.
        p.   cm. — (The Clinician's toolbox)
    Includes bibliographical references and index.
    ISBN 1-57230-105-8 (pbk.)
    1. Psychotherapy—Practice. 2. Psychotherapy—Marketing.
3. Managed mental health care. 4. Mental health consultation—
Practice. 5. Industrial psychiatry—Practice. I. Title. II. Series.
III. Series: Zuckerman, Edward L. Clinician's toolbox.
    [DNLM: 1. Practice Management, Medical—economics—United
States. 2. Fee-for-Service Plans—United States. 3. Financing,
Personal—United States. W 80 A182b 1997]
RC465.5.A25   1997
616.89′14′068—dc21
DNLM/DLC
for Library of Congress   96-48406
                                                                   CIP

To our children,
Brian, Amanda, and Pete

It is not simply your youth that gives us
hope for the future. It is your
intelligence, character, love,
and imagination.

Foreword

It is with great pleasure that I welcome Dr. Ackley's book to the Clinician's Toolbox Series of practical resources for working clinicians. *Breaking Free of Managed Care* offers you a "blueprint" for reorienting your practice for success in these stressful times. It joins other practice aids in the series: the *Clinician's Thesaurus*—for "hammering out" reports, and *The Paper Office*—the "operator's manual" for legal and ethical psychotherapy practices.

Dr. Ackley's book comes to our rescue with absolutely crucial "tools" to enable psychotherapists to flourish in an era dominated by the irrational and nonclinical constraints imposed by managed care. Like the best psychotherapy, he offers new information, an example of success (his own practice), and practical advice and guidance based on his extensive experience in adapting and helping others to adapt to the current environment. These tools are applied in three large areas: a more productive view of the practice of psychotherapy, how to market traditional psychotherapy services, and how to use your clinical skills in the workplace.

Dr. Ackley is foremost a therapist, and so he deals in Part I not with the nature of managed care or ways out of our current predicament (these are effectively addressed later), but with what is for many of us the underrated first roadblock—our pessimism and anxiety, our avoidance and escape fantasies, our passivity and helplessness. Like a fine therapist, he offers us empathy from his own painful experiences and restores our hope. He invites us to "rediscover our value" and repair the damage to our professional selves. He opens the door for those who see only the cage of managed care-controlled psychotherapy.

In Parts II and III he offers us two detailed and practical scenarios for success: marketing traditional services more effectively, and transfer-

ring our clinical skills to the work environment. Here is where Dr. Ackley's book comes to our rescue a second time. He reframes the task in
terms we all understand: taking the client's perspective ("How to Learn
from Your Market") and meeting the client's needs first ("Planning the
Business of Your Practice"). He then shows you how to effectively "Market Traditional Services."

Dr. Ackley has taken his clinical skills to the world of business and
industry. In Part III he shows us how he has accomplished this and how
he has shown other professionals the way to successful consulting relationships in the workplace. In what he calls "People-Consulting" he encourages us to use our clinical backgrounds and our "psychological
mindedness" with both workers and employers.

If you feel the need to take your independent practice into the future,
there is no better guide to that journey than this book. We all owe Dr.
Ackley a debt of gratitude for showing us the way.

—EDWARD ZUCKERMAN, PH.D.

Preface

Think of me as your scout. For 23 years I have been a therapist, but the onslaught of managed care has disrupted my practice and my sense of well-being. I imagine it has done the same to you. My initial emotional responses were similar to what most therapists tell me they experienced: denial, then depression, anxiety, and rage.

Then I took a different course. I could see that my profession was putting its entire focus on managed care: complaining, fighting, and accommodating it. I complained and fought, as well. Then I set out to search for other choices we might have. Is managed care correct in telling us that "we're the only game in town," or do *viable* alternatives exist?

Breaking Free of Managed Care is a report on the territory I am discovering. You will be pleased to know that there are abundant options that appeal to the diversity of skills and interests represented by our broad profession. No one should, or could, implement all of the practice alternatives outlined in this book.

Some of what you will read are steps I have already taken to develop a practice outside of managed care. While my own practice is in a process of transition, progress has been rapid and successful. Historically, about 10% of my practice income had been from private pay. Within 14 months of the beginning of my transition, 70%–90% (depending on the month) of my practice income was independent of any third-party reimbursement or connection. The large majority of my clients, who continue to represent a broad range of income levels, now choose to forgo their insurance "benefits." In addition, diversification of my practice into services free of insurance (and thus free of managed care) has added significantly to my income and the enjoyment of my practice.

Other ideas outlined in this book are currently being developed or tested. Some ideas come from other scouts. Some are extensions of the model that I have developed to serve as a foundation for practicing in the new territory. Finally, many ideas have come from people outside our profession. They have much to teach us.

You will be pleased to find that the choices we have are well within our behavioral range, once we achieve some shifts in our cognitive focus and learn a few new skills. You may be pleasantly surprised to find that the values in which we have long believed work better *without* third-party reimbursement than *with* it. Contrary to our fears, developing good "business of practice skills" enhances our ability to make therapy valuable. Putting the business of practice in its proper place is the fundamental tool we can use to regain our control over the ethical issues in our practices.

Breaking Free of Managed Care is a work in progress. Managed care is a new problem for us. Therefore, exploration, testing, and implementation of this model continue. I could have delayed this report until all steps were complete. However, there are three reasons it is urgent that we begin making changes now.

First, even those comfortable with managed care acknowledge that it can accommodate only 33%–50% of current therapists. Without alternatives, the majority of us will need to change jobs. Not only is that bad for us, it is bad for our society. Our society needs the services we are trained to provide.

Second, our clients need choices that go beyond what managed care is designed to offer. Managed care may be prepared to provide consultation around emotional crises and help reduce the most severe symptomatology around those crises. But, those who need other kinds of services will not get them unless we offer them outside the managed care industry. In addition, adequate privacy will not exist unless nonmanaged therapy services are available.

Third, we do not have forever to change. There is presently a window of opportunity, but that window will close for those who take too long to make adjustments. The old opportunities for practice will have evaporated and the "opportunities" offered by managed care will be closed. Those of us who do not change will then be out of business. Therefore, you need the information already gathered now!

By sharing with you what I have already discovered, you will be free to begin your own explorations from a new starting point, without having to reinvent the wheel. Then *you too* can report back on *your* scouting adventures. The more of us who are working on this, the more areas of territory we can open up for ourselves and our entire culture. It is a big task. As you will see, we are doing nothing short of redefining the relationship between our profession and our society.

Therefore, I invite you to write to me about your experiences when you finish reading and begin to put some of your ideas into practice. What steps did *you* take that worked for you? What new ideas have *you* discovered? We invite participants in our seminar, "Building a Managed Care Free Practice," to write to us, as well. And they do. We assemble their letters into a newsletter so that everyone can see the progress. Because therapists scouting this new ground are working contrary to "conventional wisdom," we need this ongoing input and support. When you write, we will share your name and ideas with others around the country. Networking opportunities will grow.

—DANA C. ACKLEY, PH.D.
3635 Manassas Drive, S.W.
Roanoke, VA 24018

Acknowledgments

Telling this story is the most challenging thing I have ever done, but no one tackles a project of this size alone. As author of this book, I am standing on the shoulders of a vast number of people. First and foremost, these shoulders belong to our colleagues, those who have created, practiced, and researched the profession of psychotherapy over the past hundred years or so, a few of whom are cited in this book. Most, however, exist within the collective unconscious of all of us. We owe them a large but payable debt. Our payment is in the protection, preservation, and extension of the value of their work.

Other shoulders I stand on belong to the hundreds of participants who have attended my seminars on "Building a Managed Care Free Practice." Through the sharing of their questions, comments, and experiences with me, the content of this book has been improved immeasurably. As mentioned in the Preface, I am a scout. Many of these professionals are scouts too and are sending their messages about ways to maintain and enhance our profession through these pages.

A third group of shoulders belongs to the Virginia Academy of Clinical Psychologists (VACP), part of the Virginia Psychological Association. VACP has a history of taking courageous stands. The Virginia Marketing Project, which I was privileged to direct, was one of those stands. It was directed toward reclaiming our profession from managed care. The membership risked time, energy, money, and reputation on a project that offered no guarantees. Many people provided key ideas, energy, and support during this project, including our Executive Secretary, Joan Smallwood, Tom DeMaio, Ph.D., Roger DeLapp, Ph.D., David Neiemeyer, Ph.D., Lee Hersch, Ph.D., and Louis A. Perrott, Ph.D. During the project, Tom and I wrote "The Dollars and Sense of Psychology in Business," a seminar script that VACP members were given to use in business presentations. Tom's dedication to getting the message about our value out to the public led him to permit me to include that material as part of our seminar handouts. Now many more therapists have access to that information. Thanks, Tom.

Many therapists have searched for ways to respond to the crisis created by managed care. At first, there was considerable unanimity of thought. We were all "against managed care." As organisms in nature mature, differentiation occurs. This is true with human organizations and movements, as well. When people move past the stage of identifying what they are against and begin to identify what they are for, differentiation naturally occurs. This book offers one differentiation.

Another perspective is that of the National Coalition of Mental Health Professionals and Consumers, Inc., led by Karen Shore, Ph.D. The goals of the Coalition are to educate professionals and the public regarding the serious problems with managed care, to work for legislative reforms to help regulate the managed care industry, and to support the development of more humane forms of third-party reimbursement. Members of the National Coalition have been extremely generous in their support of my workshops and writings even though we have different strategies in responding to managed care.

Another group, the American Mental Health Alliance, Inc., is being organized by Peter Gumpert, Ph.D. Its goal is to establish a national network of providers that will pursue direct contracts with employers.

Finally, both Janet Pipal, Ph.D., and Arthur Kovacs, Ph.D., offer seminars around the country that provide to therapists who attend their own ways of avoiding managed care. Twenty years ago we ignored Kovacs's (Kovacs & Albee, 1975) warning about the dangers of third-party reimbursement. Now his vision has proven to be on target.

You may know of other people who are attacking various aspects of our problem. While each of us is identifying different solutions, and argues for them intensely, we all continue to share an abiding concern about our profession — specifically, an awareness of what would happen to our society without the valuable services we have to offer — and an energy for alerting our society to the problems managed care presents.

Ivan Miller, Ph.D., who also is deeply involved in the National Coalition, invested a tremendous amount of time and energy in reviewing this book for publication. His comments and suggestions were extremely helpful, and he will find that I have incorporated many of them into the book. I thank him for lending his perspective and for his incredible generosity of spirit.

Ray Deveaux, Vice President of NCS Assessments, asked me to write this book for NCS. His invitation inspired me to put together a proposal. He asked me to write the book because he had seen me quoted on the value of therapy. It was a message he believed in and a message he wanted delivered to a profession in trouble. Even though I wound up going with the Guilford Press, Ray continued to support the project. In fact, his company sponsors many of my seminars, through the excellent work of Brad Ross and Kristie Everson.

Frank Taylor is a name you will find throughout this book. This insurance executive turned marketing consultant is a personal inspiration to me. He too saw the value of our contributions to society and wanted them preserved. He taught me, and others in VACP, a great deal about the potential we have for working with the business community and the mutual benefits of that work. His creative imagination about what we can do led directly to my vision of "People-Consulting in the Workplace."

I particularly want to mention Bridget Prouty, the office manager for our practice group. In the body of the work you will read why her services are so vital to the success of our practice. While she has not been directly involved in the book, her ongoing dedication to our group, the high quality of her work, and her consistently sound judgment made it possible for me to take the time necessary to put the book together.

It is hard to imagine being associated with a better publisher than the Guilford Press. Bob Matloff, President, and Seymour Weingarten, Editor-in-Chief, have offered tremendous support to this project. They saw a message they believed needed to be delivered and have worked hard with me in getting the job done. I thank Ed Zuckerman, Ph.D., for including this book in *The Clinician's Toolbox* series. Ed's input as an experienced author and fellow psychologist has been much appreciated.

Guilford's best move was asking Barbara Watkins, their editor for this book, to work with me. It has consistently amazed me how Barbara has been able make organization out of chaos. Drafts would be sent to her. They would come back with comments like "This paragraph in Chapter 8 belongs in Chapter 2." How could she keep it all straight? I couldn't. Not only that, she has significantly improved the thinking process in the book through her suggestions. She could help me see how various passages might be misunderstood and then offered significant improvements. She identified holes in logic and helped me figure out how to fill them. She also demonstrated considerable knowledge about our field. Barbara managed to provide criticisms within a context of emotional support.

You will read a lot about my partner, Louis A. Perrott, Ph.D. We have been friends and partners since 1978. Mostly we have done business on a handshake. No one ever had a more generous person as partner. We have been through many challenges together. He reviewed many sections of this book, and his comments added greatly to my perspective. But, then, they always have.

My parents, Richard and Bonnie Ackley, have been wonderful. They have consistently supported my risk taking with excitement and encouragement. They are fun to tell stories to because they listen so well. They are intelligent, reflective people to whom I owe a long standing debt of gratitude. You will meet my mother through her contribution to Chapter 8. My brother, Roger, has provided emotional support and business expertise. Many of the insights about how to sell services, how to understand the business mentality, and the ethical integrity that exists within most of the business world come from Roger. He has been a role model in more ways than he knows.

Finally, the most important person in this whole project is my wife, Peg. She is the smartest person I know, and the sweetest. She has contributed many of the ideas not only in the book but also in the seminar. She carefully listens to presentations to help with logic and with presentation style. She shares the excitement of the message. Within the past year she has joined me in working full time to get our message delivered. Our profession will be the better for her contributions.

Beyond that, I have needed her loving support particularly over the past few years. I can imagine many spouses who would have panicked at the thought of the risks we are taking. Peg never flinched. I remember telling her about managed care and my unwillingness to participate. "Of course, you can't," she said. Fearing that she did not fully appreciate the situation and needing to share my own despair, I told her, "You don't understand. I could lose my practice. We would lose our house. We'll be poor. . . . " Her basic response was, "So?" Thanks, Peg.

Contents

PART I

LOOKING BEYOND MANAGED CARE

People who practice psychotherapy are about to become the preeminent professionals of the twenty-first century.

As a psychotherapist, how do you react to this statement? Do you find it ludicrous? Everyone seems to predict our profession's demise. There are new reasons to be discouraged everywhere. Services to clients are increasingly restricted. Autonomy is disappearing, and income is dwindling. Professional organizations tell us to get with the managed care program or plan to park cars for a living. Managed care *then* tells us that it can use only about one-third of the therapists currently in practice. Is it any wonder that we are depressed, going out of business, or both? And we are supposed to help people feel better?!

How can a rational person claim we are about to enter a period of preeminence? As Milton Erickson showed us, focus is everything. When people are focused on their limits and disabilities, they are limited and disabled. Our profession's entire focus is currently on managed care. Go to any professional meeting. Read any journal. There it is. Even before we saw it coming, managed care grabbed our income stream, a sure way to command someone's attention. In response, we have become transfixed, even hypnotized. Like spotlighted deer, we became so focused on one aspect of reality that other parts have slipped into the background unnoticed. We have forgotten to remember our value, the foundation of our strength and opportunity. Forgetting our value has led us to make decisions antithetical not only to our own well being but to our clients' as well.

Our *potential* value has not changed because of the rise of managed

1

care. We *are* in danger, however, of letting that value become eroded if managed care continues to dominate how therapy is delivered. This eventuality would be a disaster for both us and our society. It is not too late to regain control of the way we practice, especially if we act now. Regaining control involves shifting our focus *away* from managed care and *toward* the elements that create our value. On that basis we can build new ways to relate to our society that preserve and expand the best of what we are and what we do.

The function of *Breaking Free of Managed Care* is to show you how to make these adjustments. It shows how you can develop a private pay practice, just as other professionals such as attorneys, CPAs, and dentists have always done. It will help you to rediscover the value of your work, discard assumptions that might block your progress, find new ways to invite people to use your services, learn reasonable business of practice skills, and build a safety net by diversifying your practice. As you put your new knowledge to work, you will be able to make stronger contributions to society and secure a good future, both for yourself and for our profession. It will require lots of hard work, but most of us are working hard anyway, with little reward for our efforts.

Rather than being a disaster, the intrusion of managed care may actually provide a wonderful opportunity. It has forced us out of our comfort zone. As long as we are uncomfortable anyway, let's look at ourselves with a new eye. When we take a hard look at who we are and what we do, we can find ways to end our dependence on third-party reimbursement and move to self-reliance. Is this so different from what we often ask of our clients?

Chapter 1

Descent, Recovery, and Our Future

The model presented in this book began its development within my own depressed and rageful reaction to what promised to be the destruction of my clinical practice. Many of you are likely to find the early part quite familiar.

MY OWN STORY

My Descent

When the 1990s began, I had 15 years of successful private practice as a clinical psychologist under my belt. Demand for my services was high. I dealt with the typical difficulties family therapists handle: school adjustment problems, marital issues, family conflicts, divorce, job stress. My referrals came from the usual sources: guidance counselors, school principals, pediatricians, family physicians, satisfied former clients, and word of mouth. Some people came for a short series of appointments, others stayed an intermediate amount of time, while still others spent years making visits. I usually had a waiting list for appointments.

My partner, Louis A. Perrott, Ph.D., and I enjoyed strong reputations in the community. Because of those reputations, other therapists asked to join us. Eventually we became the Manassas Group, one of the largest outpatient practice groups in southwestern Virginia, with 15 therapists representing four therapy professions. We created a niche for ourselves with uncompromising quality, diversity of service, strong secretarial/receptionist support, and attractive facilities.

My three children, a new house, pets, and the other adornments of a middle-class lifestyle depended on a steady, growing income. While not outrageous, the income my practice generated was quite good. This sense of financial dependability encouraged me to deny that the growing cloud of managed care would actually cross my horizon.

This pattern of denial was shattered in October 1991, when a letter arrived from one of the leaders of my state professional organization, the Virginia Academy of Clinical Psychologists (VACP). The letter reported that our state's largest health insurer had teamed up with a huge managed care company. Until then, I had never even heard of that company, and now, suddenly, it seemed all consuming. The vision of this duo taking over mental health care in our state was vivid. While this particular partnership never achieved the full force of my fantasies, it signaled the beginning of the end of indemnity insurance, the bedrock of my financing structure. As other managed care companies began feeding on the businesses in our state, the collapse of my practice was easy to picture.

I began to realize that the financial success of my practice was no longer guaranteed. My competence and caring for my clients were no longer enough. My ability to control my future seemed to evaporate. Control now rested in other hands. Those hands belonged to people who did not know me and who had no reason to have any interest in my well-being. It was like any trauma. The fantasy of safety, which we all use to get through the day, was unceremoniously ripped away, revealing the true dangers of the world. From all sides came the warning that the only safe path was to "play ball" with the new order.

The Manassas Group met with the managed care company mentioned in the denial-shattering letter. We discussed joining their provider panel. The meeting was intensely upsetting. These people *seriously* expected episodes of care to run about six sessions. They provided sample treatment protocols that looked *nothing* like what I did. They seemed so sure that this was *the right way* to practice that I began to question seriously my approach to therapy.

If they could get the results they claimed in so few sessions, what was wrong with me? Had I been incompetent? Had I allowed myself to keep people in treatment too long just to serve my needs? Had I been in the bathroom when someone found the cure to mental illness? Managed care seemed to think so.

After considering my options, I did the only thing I could envision: I became deeply depressed and acutely anxious. My sleep was interrupted with visions of being out of work and of the shame of being exposed as a bad therapist. I became impatient with clients whose pattern of change did not match the expectations of my new authority figures.

Although I did not apply to join any managed care provider panels,

I did begin filling out outpatient treatment reports (OTRs) and doing phone utilization review (UR) reports for clients who saw me "out of panel." These experiences contributed to my distress. The managed care approach to treatment, heavily based on the medical model, forced me to describe my work in terms ill suited to my approach. The concepts managed care seemed to value had rarely been of much use to me when I was actually in the room with a human being. I certainly had studied psychopathology in graduate school and beyond, and many have considered me to be an excellent diagnostician. Yet, over the years I had found it more efficacious to focus on strengths and resources than on disease categories.

Maybe, I thought, that is my problem. Maybe I have been ignoring the things I should have been paying attention to. In doing the UR reviews, I had to submerge my real concerns and interests in deference to the concerns of managed care. With only so much time available with clients, I seemed to be devoting an awful lot of it to what was wrong, not to what was useful. It was demoralizing and, I felt, unfair to the people who came to see me.

For some time I whined, moaned, cried, and predicted personal disaster. There was no shortage of sob sisters. After a while, however, it became apparent that this "strategy" was not helping much. No one outside my profession cared about my pitiful complaints. Even my family eventually grew weary of them. Meanwhile, the power of managed care continued to build as my self-esteem proceeded in its self-destruction. Managed care challenged my self-esteem, it challenged my professional integrity, and it challenged my financial self-sufficiency.

Bottoming Out

Change was being forced on me. The question, I discovered, was not *whether* my practice would change but *who* would direct that change— myself or someone else? At first, I was too immobolized by depression, anxiety, and rage to direct change. I could not decide what to do, especially because all of the choices I could see at the time seemed so awful. I looked hard at trying to join preferred provider panels. It would have meant earning 30% less while working longer hours filling out useless paperwork and begging for sessions reviewers did not want to give to people who needed them. I would have to practice in ways that I believed to be substandard, while my clients would get only those restricted services managed care was willing to provide. One highly competent, well-established therapist echoed my mood at the time: "What else can we do?"

During my period of immobilization, it felt like outside, unfriendly forces would be shaping my future. Managed care was essentially running a want ad that said:

Help wanted: Therapists

Lower pay!
Longer hours!
Lower quality!
Less autonomy!

It was really scary when that began to look attractive. It scared me enough to take action.

My Ascent

Because of the strong emphasis on research in our graduate programs, clinical psychologists are trained to look at data. It finally dawned on me that I had not examined the data on our clinical and cost effectiveness. I had assumed managed care knew what it was talking about. The assumption was wrong.

I looked at the data. The more I looked, the better I felt. By reading the next chapter, you can look too. You will find that, as a group, outpatient therapists have always been clinically effective *and* cost-effective.

The data demonstrate that the claims made by managed care are not based on reality. For example, VACP commissioned a review of the literature (Kiesler & Wagner, 1992) that a major managed care company used to justify its six session approach. The reviewers were experienced researchers in therapy. Their review concluded that the purported "justification" for a six-session model was in fact based on a cursory examination of an outdated and inadequate collection of studies. The fact that managed care had convinced so many buyers otherwise did not make their claims true. This knowledge, based on the Kiesler and Wagner review and the extensive literature to be considered in the next chapter, led me to a decision that I had wrestled with since getting the letter. I would not join managed care.

I knew that my decision could cost me my practice and my family's livelihood. Doing what you believe to be right does not guarantee survival. However, both my way of practicing and my personality were fundamentally unsuited to managed care. For me it would have been wrong to join. If that meant having to change how I made my living, I would have to face that. My partner and I developed a standing joke about finding a golf course to run. Not a bad way to live, actually.

But I did not want to quit my profession. My interest in doing therapy began in early adolescence. Like most teens, I experimented mentally with a variety of alternatives. I always came home. It is how I have spent my adult life.

My choice to leave the profession, if it came to that, rather than join managed care, had a welcome but unexpected effect. It brought me great relief. I no longer felt at the mercy of others. I realized that I would control my fate, one way or another. The illusion that others were in control of my future was self imposed. The relief allowed me to think clearly, which was critical to finding ways to *stay* in my profession.

Over the next several years, I researched and experimented with ways of responding to managed care. The first thought, having looked at the data on therapy outcome and cost effectiveness, was to share this information with the business community. It seemed reasonable to suppose that, if they knew the truth, they would abandon managed care and go back to an indemnity approach that paid improved attention to mental health issues.

Several local professional groups worked together to put on a presentation of the data to our local business community. I got to make the presentation. It went so well that the VACP asked me to head up a statewide program. This program eventually became known as the Virginia Marketing Project and became a model that other professional groups across the nation worked with. The project never achieved the goals I had for it; yet it was an extremely useful experience. The relevant lessons will be shared with you as we work through this book.

As a natural extension of my experience with the Virginia Marketing Project, I began to consider direct contracting with businesses. Basically, this would have involved joining with other therapists to set up our own managed care company. The hope was that, because we understood the therapy process and the needs of clients, we could do a more humane job of managing care and retain control of our practices. At the same time, we could still save employers money because of the greater cost effectiveness of good outpatient therapy.

However, I realized that therapist-owned managed care companies would face the same financial pressures as their competitors. To be able to compete on price, they too would have to find ways to restrict costs. This eventually would lead to limits on services and fees because those factors account for the lion's share of the costs. The pressure would still be there to achieve rapid results at the expense of taking the time needed by the client.

Further, I noticed that marketplace issues could also put therapist-owned companies in jeopardy. First, well-capitalized managed care companies can "buy business" until competitors with less capital can no longer survive. A well-funded company can choose to lose money on contracts for a year or two as an investment in the long term. This means they sell services for less than it costs to provide them. When companies with less money in the bank try to compete on price, they are the ones who run out of money first. Therapist-owned companies that do not compete on price are vulnerable to being cut out of contracts.

Second, I could picture our spending the time and capital necessary to create such a company—only to fall victim to the health care field's evolution in directions that would make our company irrelevant! Health care is going through a process of rapid evolution. The next generation of managed care will provide services through "fully integrated health care delivery systems." These "one-stop shopping" health care companies are designed to provide everything a health care purchaser (i.e., an employer) might want, from health insurance and benefit design, to outpatient medical services, hospital care, catastrophic care, and *mental health services*. They can accurately be described as vertically integrated *monopolies*.

To illustrate, health care in our area is now dominated by two huge health care organizations, each of which owns a growing number of hospitals and specialty clinics. One of them has been buying a large number of physicians' private practices, turning those physicians into employees. (Mental health providers' practices have not been purchased. Those providers have simply been hired.) The other company is closely associated with a 145-member physician group. Each organization offers local employers a wide array of services, including mental health services, on a capitated basis, and is able to offer volume discounts because of economies of scale—well beyond what could be offered by small groups or even large groups-without-walls. One of these companies has also formed a strategic partnership with a large health insurance company in our state to enhance the package they offer. That insurance company has changed some of its advertising and now calls itself a health care company.

Gayle Tuttle, editor of *Practice Strategies,* predicts that similar monoliths will swallow up most of the mental health carve out companies currently dominating the market (private communication, 1995). Workshops given during the American Psychological Association's Leadership Training Conferences (Bachman, 1995) tend to support this prediction. To be players in the new managed care arena, therapists will either have to be owners of the megacorporations or employed by them. Preferred provider panels will be a thing of the past. This is important information for those of us considering opening our own managed care companies. It is also important information for therapists who have joined panels in order to stay in practice. That financing structure is likely to evaporate as has our old friend, indemnity insurance.

As employers turn to these health care companies for benefit management, employees wishing to access their health insurance to pay for therapy will have to see a therapist employed by the health care company. Employees who pay out of pocket will be able to see any independent therapist they choose, *provided there are any left.*

Third, as I explored these options, I found myself responding to issues that managed care companies and insurance companies wanted to highlight. It eventually dawned on me that their issues are not my issues. So long as I stayed focused on their issues, my thinking was limited. When I began letting go of their issues, I could begin to see the problems we face in a different light and develop other solutions.

We need alternatives that put *us* in control of the services we provide. The problem with *any* form of third-party reimbursement is that it maintains dependence on other people's money. Because people like to control what they pay for, third-party payers will *always* want to intrude on our relationship with our clients. It is not unreasonable for them to do so. Don't you want to control how *your* money is spent?

One reason to tell this story is that so much of it is common to all of us—the love of the profession, the current terror, depression, self-doubt, and the questions about what to do. A more important reason is that these experiences propelled me on a course of discovery that I believe provides real hope for our profession. Though I didn't realize my ultimate destination at the time, the letter I received in 1991 started me toward the development of a model of a managed care free practice. I am using this model for my own practice, but I can see it broadly applied to our entire profession. Over the past five years, I have found a rich range of alternatives to managed care. These alternatives represent the wonderful diversity our profession offers.

LOOKING BEYOND MANAGED CARE

If you are thinking about pursuing a managed care free practice, I must warn you that just making the decision to stay outside of managed care is not enough. To be successful, you will need a conceptual framework to guide your decision making in this new endeavor. This framework is different in some ways from the one we have used for the past 20 years. You will also need to develop business of practice skills most of us have lacked. You will have to know the real reasons we got into trouble, which are quite different from the reasons put forth by managed care. Interestingly, many therapists who have heard the conceptual framework outlined in my seminars on "Building a Managed Care Free Practice" report that it fits precisely with ideas that they have long valued but that have little acceptance in the current marketplace.

Yet, you may find that the needed conceptual shifts are difficult to make. Internal shifts in assumptions are hard to make while we are transfixed by external factors. Assumptions are notoriously hard for people to identify because they are so embedded in our behavior and psyches. One assumption that most of us have made is that third-party reimbursement is essential to a successful outpatient practice. "Everyone" knows that. What if "everyone" is wrong? *Our current predicament rests entirely upon our dependence on third-party reimbursement. If we remove that dependence, the power of managed care is gone.* To most of us, letting go of third-party reimbursement has been unthinkable. Because it has been inconceivable, we have made some compromises in how we practice. We made compromises for the sake of providing truncated services, believing them to be better than no services at all. This belief is questionable.

If we really want control of our practices, the only alternative I can see is direct payment by those who use our services. While this may seem like an impossible dream, my experience shows that clients are far more ready for this approach than you may believe. Furthermore, its benefits are compellingly superior for both you *and* your clients. Control of the therapy process returns to the two people best qualified to make judgments about it. You and your client are free to establish a relationship that fits the client's needs rather than those of a third party. As this book unfolds, you will learn why your clients, like mine, will decide it is worth the money.

The services available under managed care are extremely limited. Our clients need other options. Short-term, symptom-oriented treatment works for some people and should be used when you and your client agree to it. Research that will be reviewed in the next chapter tells us exactly when to use such methods. It also shows that we do not need to be managed to use short-term treatment when appropriate. However, other clients have other needs. We must have ways to fill those needs, too.

> She was an angry, lonely woman. She complained of great distress. Her sleep was lousy. She had little fun, few social connections, and she trusted no one. Suicidal thoughts were frequent. She felt "just awful." She hated her job even though she had worked hard to win the advanced degree it required. Actually, she did not like any job that she had any longer than a few months.
>
> Slowly her story came out. She was raised by an alcoholic mother who likely was intermittently psychotic. Physical and verbal abuse were ever-present threats and frequent realities. Her parents had loud, frightening fights with regularity. Whereas her older siblings learned what many learn in alcoholic families, to keep their mouths shut, she made different decisions as a child. She sometimes asked questions and complained, even though it was dangerous. As an adult, in other settings, she sometimes spoke up when it was not appropriate and did not speak up when she should have.
>
> She saw me for 5 years, sometimes weekly but more often every 2 weeks because that was the frequency that worked best for her. Intermittently, especially as I sweated about managed care, I wor-

ried that she had come too long. At one point, she made a statement that put it in perspective for me: "Dana, I spent an entire childhood in that crazy family. My whole adult life I have been living with the residue. I do not think that 130 hours in this room is an excessive amount of time to recover from that."

Her therapy did eventually come to an end, though not before her insurance quit paying. She chose to pay out of pocket and continue because it was valuable to her to do so. The outcome was that she felt much better. Her anger was manageable and expressed effectively when needed. She felt good about herself. She slept well. Her social life blossomed. She changed jobs within her field of expertise, gaining a position worthy of her. Could these outcomes have occurred under short-term therapy? She and I do not think so. Were the services "medically necessary"? We don't care. They were valuable to her, and she paid for them.

It is not appropriate to keep people in therapy that has no ongoing value. However, there are many good reasons for people to have long-term therapy. This woman's story illustrates just some of those reasons. Our clients need alternatives to short-term therapy, and we must be prepared to provide them.

Our society is beginning to discover that paying attention to psychological and emotional issues can have great benefits, but this understanding is still fragile. There are still too many ways that psychological ignorance causes destruction. We can help society only if we maintain the integrity of who we are, what we do, and what makes it valuable.

THE MISSION OF THIS BOOK

My mission is to provide us with the conceptual and practical tools required to reengineer our practices to operate outside the third-party reimbursement system. Achieving the necessary changes entails five steps:

1. Restoring our sense of professional self-esteem and integrity by rediscovering our value.
2. Reconceptualizing some of the fundamental assumptions by which we organize our practices.
3. Learning basic business skills to protect our practices.
4. Learning how to develop the private pay market for traditional therapy and assessment services.
5. Diversifying our services, that is, learning new applications for what we already know. In this book, "People-Consulting in the Workplace" will be the primary illustration.

The rest of this book examines these five steps in detail, providing a map for you to follow. Chapters 2–4 focus on giving you the conceptual tools needed to act. Reading these chapters will help to restore your professional self-esteem and will remind you of the true value of what you offer. Do we see people too long or charge too much? When we look at the data, we will see that the financial benefits far outweigh the costs for our services. But third-party payment and its use of the medical model have gradually distorted the way we organize our practices. We need to reexamine our basic assumptions and reconceptualize our practices in accord with our true value and what people really want. When we do this, opportunities and options that have been hard to see become clearly visible.

If we are to take advantage of these opportunities, however, we must face the emotionally difficult issues of money and business honestly and squarely. In coming to terms with the fact that we *are* in business, we can begin to see that our traditional lack of business skills has put us at the mercy of others who do not have our psychological skills. To regain control of our practices and maintain our ethics, we must acquire the tools of business and use them honorably. You will find this to be more feasible than you might at first imagine.

With this foundation, we can begin to act. Chapters 5–8 teach the basic business skills you need to develop a private pay practice. These skills include creating a business plan and marketing your services successfully. We also look at the practicalities of making the transition from a third-party dependent practice to one that is managed care free. Chapters 9–12 help you to create a safety net for your practice. They explain how you can diversify the services you offer by learning new applications for what you already know.

The tools you will find in this book will provide an alternative to losing control of your practice to large, impersonal bureaucracies. You will learn how to preserve and extend the value of therapy while making managed care *irrelevant* to your own practice.

Chapter 2

Restoring Professional Self-Esteem, Rediscovering Our Value

Our dependence upon third-party reimbursement set us up for a psychological problem. As we counted increasingly on insurance money to support us, we began unconsciously to allow our sense of worth to be tied to the willingness of insurance companies to pay us. When those companies began to question the value of paying us, we began to question the worth of our services, and, for many of us, our self-esteem began to erode. Our cognitions became distorted. Some may believe that we can reestablish our self-respect by returning to the old style of third-party reimbursement. That is never going to happen. Fortunately, there is a more effective foundation available for our self-respect.

The simple truth is that what we do has empirically supported value. That value can be seen and measured in dollar terms and beyond. Examining the research on the value and cost-effectiveness of traditional psychotherapy reestablished my sense of competence. It also renewed my faith in the ethics I brought to my practice. I believe it will have similar effects on yours, as well. All of us who decide to swim upstream against conventional wisdom, as this book invites you to do, will inevitably experience severe doubts from time to time. These data help provide needed reassurance that we are on the right track. I invite you to spend some time reviewing the effectiveness of your profession. Contrast what you read with the myths created about us by managed care. In this chapter we will first identify those myths and the reasons why managed care created them. Then we will look at the data that demolish them.

HOW MANAGED CARE SOLD ITSELF
TO EMPLOYERS

We can all agree that health care costs were getting out of hand. We certainly have heard it often enough in the news, and our own health care premiums are monthly reminders. The extent to which people experience rising health care costs depends on the extent to which they actually pay for their own health care services. The people who care the most about these rising costs are employers, because they are the ones who are paying most of them, through employee benefit plans. With businesses having trouble containing health care costs, it was only a matter of time before someone came up with a solution. That's how the free market system works. Enter managed care.

Managed care officials looked at the categories of health care to find out where the costs were concentrated. Then they proceeded to cut costs. When they got to outpatient mental health costs, they found that the average number of sessions per episode of care was between 6 and 8. Only 9.8% of episodes of care lasted longer than 25 sessions. However, that 9.8% of episodes consumed 50% of outpatient therapy costs. (Taube, Keeler, & Feuerberg, 1984, cited by Bak, Weiner, & Jackson, 1991).

Managed care officials realized that, based on cost considerations alone, they could dramatically reduce outpatient mental health costs right away by eliminating episodes that run past 25 sessions. And so they did. (How often have you heard something like, "Your patient's benefit package does not pay for long-term therapy"?) To control costs further, they determined to have people use no more than that average of 6–8 sessions. This step was intended to yield predictability of costs, something that had been missing. In many ways, predictability of costs is more important to businesses than absolute cost, because the pricing for a company's products may be adjusted so long as costs can be accurately predicted. Employers' greatest anxiety about health care costs has been that, under the old fee-for-service model, no one seemed able to predict costs with any reasonable accuracy.

Cost-cutting decisions based on these statistics alone are, of course, shortsighted. We will see that the net value of sessions beyond the average of 6–8, even beyond 25, is greater than the original cost outlay. *But that may not matter to decision makers.* In today's fast-paced business environment, taking the farsighted view is often not a practical alternative for decision makers. Chief executive officers and business opportunities come and go so rapidly that it is often all one can do to make a profit *today.* If costs are cut and profits go up on *their* watch, that is enough for many CEOs. Problems that may result as a consequence in the future will be *someone else's* challenge.

Well aware of employers' mindset and priorities, the managed care industry marketed mental health products to them by making two accusations about outpatient therapists, namely, that we keep people in therapy too long and charge too much for it. These claims support managed care's financial and marketing goals, but are they true? Are they supported by the data? Without understanding the climate in which many business decisions are made today, it is easy to conclude that managed care's decision to jettison therapy as we know it had to do with its intrinsic and economic value. But let's look at the facts.

EXPLODING MYTHS ABOUT PSYCHOTHERAPY

Do We Really See People Too Long? What the Data Show

The question of therapy's ideal duration is far more complex than the marketing messages used by managed care have led many to believe. Despite the dire warnings that outpatient therapy was growing out of control, VandenBos (personal communication, March 20, 1992) notes that outpatient therapy has accounted for 3%–4% of the nation's total health care bill every quarter of every year since 1977. In other words, there has been no explosion of outpatient therapy costs. This information is based on the quarterly reports from the Health Service and Research Administration of the Federal Government, which monitors health care spending patterns.

I decided to look at the average length of episodes of care in my own practice. Mentally focused only on those clients who came to see me for a long time, I expected a very high average. I was wrong. My average is 13 sessions per episode of care. It is probably higher than the national average because of a much smaller percentage of one- and two-session episodes. According to Bak, Weiner, and Jackson (1991), 48% of outpatient episodes of care consist of only one or two visits. Therapists successful in private practice have probably learned relationship-building skills that serve to keep people around long enough for them to get results.

Managed care did not consider why the average number of sessions was so low and whether there might be clinical and cost benefits for more sessions. This would have interfered with their goal of looking for a short term solution to employers' cost problems.

The core question, at least for us, is: Do clinical benefits justify the expense of extended treatment? We need to separate this question from the question of what business is willing to pay for. If business decides it must take a short-term view, there is nothing we can do. It is their money and their choice. But this choice has little to do with our value.

Clinical Benefits and Length of Treatment

The question of clinical benefit is basically the *dose/effect* question, an increasingly prominent area of psychotherapy outcome research. Such research parallels drug-based research that examines how the size of the dosage of a particular drug affects the drug's impact on the patient's condition. When applied to psychotherapy, dose/effect studies examine whether the size of the dose (number of sessions) is related to the size of the effect (outcome). If there is no advantage to having more sessions, then there is no reason to provide them. However, if there are genuine benefits, then extending the length of treatment is indicated. This is a much more useful criterion than one based solely on cost.

Herron, Javler, Primavera, and Schultz (1994), Howard, Kopta, Krause, and Orlinsky (1986), and McNally and Howard (1991) examined the dose/effect research. The studies they cite show that large gains often do occur early in treatment, often within the first 6–8 sessions. Studies further show that 75% of clients improve within 26 sessions. This conclusion could argue for a managed care approach to therapy—unless, of course, you happen to be in the 25% that needs more than 26 sessions. In addition, this conclusion does not consider whether improvement continues beyond the initial gains. In other words, after the initial gains, can more gains be made? Finally, this research did not look at whether gains are maintained posttreatment.

Steenbarger (1994) went the next step in his meta-analysis of therapy outcome studies. His key contribution was to consider how researchers defined improvement. He found that most studies defined improvement in one of two ways, either as symptom improvement or as trait change. Understanding how researchers variously define outcomes clears up much of the confusion in the literature.

Steenbarger looked at a number of variables as they relate to outcome. He first looked at duration of treatment. The studies he reviewed show that it is relatively easy to get rapid symptom improvement. However, it takes a lot more time to achieve trait change. Thus, if the definition of "improvement" is a matter of symptoms, short-term therapy looks pretty good. For people looking to make more basic changes in themselves, perhaps to ward off the likelihood of having another bout of symptoms, brief therapy does not do as well as longer-term therapy. More time in therapy is required to change traits than managed care usually allows.

What Steenbarger found in the research literature seems to conform to what most practicing clinicians have always known on the basis of their clinical judgment and observations. If someone has spent a lifetime building a personality pattern, changing the pattern itself takes more time than countering the latest instances of symptomatic behavior.

Steenbarger found similar results with respect to type of therapy offered. His review shows that brief, symptom-focused therapies do better than dynamically oriented therapies in achieving the kind of rapid symptom-oriented changes that managed care defines as "medically necessary." However, longer-term dynamic therapies do better at effecting deeper personality change.

Again, this observation makes clinical common sense. Brief therapy is *designed* to treat symptoms—hence, it is not too surprising that it does a better job. Conversely, dynamically oriented therapy is *oriented* to more fundamental aspects of personality, and thus it is not surprising that it does a better job with them. The research shows that schools of therapy do what they are intended to do.

In my own practice, clients often experience rapid symptom reduction. For some, that is all they want, and they go on their way. Many, however, choose to stay to examine themselves more deeply. In those situations, the therapy approach then shifts from symptom-oriented techniques to methods better suited to long-term work. Most of my colleagues report similar practice patterns.

Steenbarger found five additional variables that mediate the relationship between duration and outcome. I predict you will find few surprises when you compare these results with your own clinical experiences.

1. *Clients who enter therapy with strong interpersonal skills achieve results faster than clients whose interpersonal skills are weak.* Those people with weak interpersonal skills need much more time just to establish a therapeutic alliance. Whereas people diagnosed as anxious or depressed showed improvement between sessions 8–13, people identified as borderline personalities needed 26–52 sessions to show similar improvement.

Consider your own experience. If it is like mine, you have some clients who come in and establish an appropriate working relationship with ease. Their histories include reliable and enduring relationships with friends and family. They begin moving toward their goals more quickly than people who come in with histories that include few enduring relationships. For these people, those relationships that have endured are characterized by exploitation and abuse. It is not surprising that these people initially put less faith in our interventions. They need those 26–52 sessions just to find out if we can be trusted.

2. *Clients actively involved in therapy change faster than those who take a more passive approach.* Active involvement is defined as emotional activation within sessions and doing one's homework.

Most therapists learn that people must change at their own speed. This is how we come to appreciate that therapy models work less well in the real world than in textbooks. Some people accept the therapist's offer of techniques and tools for rapid change. They get actively involved in the process, while the therapist's main job is to stay out of the way. Other people resist. The resistance has important meaning, and little change will occur until that resistance is both considered and overcome. This is "Therapy 101." Yet, I hear stories of clients' resistance being ignored because it does not fit the short-term model under which therapists are now constrained to act. Slow changers need support during the time they require for change. People are unable to alter their fundamental personality to suit someone else's psychological model.

3. *When presenting problems are clearly defined, it takes less time in therapy to achieve the desired results. When the presenting problems are complex or vague, therapy takes longer to achieve positive outcomes.* People able to articulate their concerns clearly are likely to be able to think about them more productively than those whose thoughts are more muddled. Muddled thinking may be an inherent part of the problem. If so, we must not only handle the presenting symptoms but also help the person learn to think more clearly. That takes a bit of time.

> The first session ended. Surprisingly to me, the client rescheduled. I thought we had not connected. The session seemed to ramble, and every time I thought I knew where we were going, he let me know I had missed it. When we got to goal setting, he used only the vaguest of terms—"to be happier." As we became better acquainted, I came to realize that this is just the way he thinks. He was not going to respond to my collection of rapid-fire techniques. If I were going to be of assistance, I would need to start where he was, not where I wanted him to be.

4. *Therapeutic gains can be lost posttreatment when contextual issues are not considered.* For example, poor marital relationships often undermine treatment gains. It is not uncommon for people to make rapid progress in their symptoms. However, if their symptoms stem from a flawed marriage, repairing those flaws helps to reduce the likelihood that those symptoms will come back. This, of course, supports the long tradition therapists have had of attending to related issues, along with the presenting problem. Therapists are not just keeping people in therapy for their own self-enrichment. They are cementing treatment gains. The research bears out our clinical judgment.

David Barlow (1991), a leading researcher on therapy for anxiety disorders, finds similar results in his research on treating anxiety. He notes that people with simple (quite rare) panic disorders respond within 8–12 sessions. People complaining of both panic disorders and related issues take longer to achieve good and lasting results.

5. *As many as 78% of short-term therapy clients who are then maintained by medication alone relapse. Their symptoms come back* (Steen-

burger, 1994). Yet, this treatment regimen has been the model that managed care seems so often to endorse. The model achieves its goals of short-term treatment at the expense of missing the original goal of lasting clinical benefit. In other words, the Golden Rule comes into play: "He who has the gold rules." The treatment goal of the payer, that treatment be short-term, is met. The treatment goal of the client gets lost.

Steenbarger's conclusion is consistent with other research reported by Barlow (1991). He found that relief from anxiety is achieved rapidly with minor tranquilizers. However, the problems generally return. In other words, people get better faster on medication. They just do not stay better. The relapse rate for people who achieve gains through Barlow's well-structured therapy program is much lower.

Antonuccio, Danton, and DeNelsky (1995) offer outstanding evidence consistent with what Steenbarger and Barlow report. In their meta-analysis of research on the treatment of depression, they examined extensive literature regarding the relative effectiveness of therapy versus antidepressant medication. Contrary to conventional wisdom, research shows that talk therapy is at least as effective as medication but without the dangerous side effects. In addition clients on medication have lower compliance, higher dropout rates, and much higher relapse rates than people who engage in talk therapy. In other words, therapy is as effective in the long run as medications, and it is safer. Finally, Antonuccio et al. found that adding medication to therapy does not improve overall outcomes.

They go on to make another interesting point. They ask, given the data, how medications became the treatment of choice. Among other factors, they note that drug companies market their product. Therapists have not.

Finally, a landmark study done by *Consumer Reports,* "Mental Health: Does Therapy Help?" (1995), determined the value of therapy from a different perspective: they asked consumers. They asked real people about their experiences in the real world. Whereas the vast majority of research reviewed by Herron (1994), Steenbarger (1994), and Antonuccio et al. (1995) was laboratory based, the *Consumer Reports* work was a naturalistic study. In constructing their survey, and in interpreting its results, the authors relied on consultation from Martin Seligman, former director of training in clinical psychology at the University of Pennsylvania. Seligman (1996) believes this study to be the best assessment of the impact of therapy on real people ever done.

Basically, the 4000 readers who responded reported that therapy helped and it helped a lot. Ninety percent of those who reported that they had begun therapy feeling "very poor" reported that therapy helped "a lot" (54%) or "somewhat" (36%). People with longer periods of treatment reported more progress than those with shorter periods. Specifically, 33% of those in therapy for 6 months or less reported that they were helped a lot, while 50% of those who stayed longer than 6 months said they were helped a lot.

This study, like the Antonuccio et al. review, compared talk therapy and drug therapy. Readers who used only talk therapy did as well as those who took drugs but without the risk of side effects. It was bothersome to note that 40% of people taking antianxiety drugs had been on them for more than a year, despite the serious risk of habituation to such medications.

In summary, a growing body of powerful research tells us what we clinicians experience on a daily basis in our offices. What we do has value. What we do works. Taking time is often necessary. The notion that a "fast-food" approach to therapy is just as effective as high-quality work is debunked.

Steenbarger's review of therapy outcome research shows that, for clients who are motivated, who define problems in clear, uncomplicated terms, and who only want symptom relief and are willing to do homework, brief therapy is the treatment of choice. If the situation is more complicated, treatment will take longer. The other studies support these conclusions. These practice patterns happen naturally, without outside management. Most therapists had done a good job of measuring and delivering what clients need before managed care.

Goals of Outpatient Therapy

Steenbarger (1994) showed us that the answer to the question "Do we keep people in therapy too long?" rests upon how we define improvement. Managed care has taken the most conservative definition of outcome available and uses it as their measure of "medical necessity." This is unsurprising since this approach offers the greatest reduction in the immediate cost of outpatient therapy.

Actually, the term "medical necessity" is misleading. It implies that there is consensus among professionals about what is necessary to treat emotional problems. The implication is that if what one is doing is not "medically necessary," it is somehow suspect. "Medical necessity" is an insurance term, not a clinical term. It was developed to provide administrative guidance, not to solve human problems. We need to accept the fact that consensus is not a strong point of our profession. This is not the weakness some claim it to be. It is important that we maintain a wide variety of ideas and treatment approaches to fit the wide variety of problems that exist and the wide variety of people who have them. The sometimes sharp disagreements that we have also lead to ongoing advances in the ways we work with people. Without the tension created by our disagreements, we might never search for or try out new ideas.

In reality, the question is not one of medical necessity, but rather a question of values. As a society we seem to agree that it is wrong to withhold medical care that is necessary. But once we move out of the area of immediate life-threatening situations, people naturally begin to disagree about what is necessary. The questions then become: What is necessary? What is important? What would be nice? The debate on these questions becomes especially heated when one group wants to spend another group's money.

Herron et al. (1994) offer a conceptualization that enables us to understand the question of length of therapy in terms of values. They suggest that outpatient therapy inherently offers goals at three levels: (1) necessity, (2) improvement, and (3) potentiality.

Necessity. At this level, treatment is designed to get rid of symptoms that keep the client from taking care of basic life functions. Typical goals of necessity treatment include having the individual meet all minimum requirements at work, keeping his or her family intact, and having reasonable hygiene. For example, a clinical depression so severe that a person seriously contemplates suicide would be treated. Once the person is no longer suicidal, necessity therapy ends. For people who experience severe anxiety that prevents them from working, treatment is aimed at returning them to the job.

Necessity-level treatment is crisis oriented and aimed at symptoms. When the crisis ends, so does treatment. You may notice that this model is similar to benefits offered under many managed care programs. In other words, it is this level of care that is usually defined as "medically necessary."

Improvement. Improvement-level goals include and build on the necessity-level ones. They take a "better than" rather than a "good enough" approach. If an individual is so depressed as to be suicidal, improvement-level treatment, like necessity-level, first insures safety. But then improvement treatment attends to the reasons for the depression. These issues are considered so that they do not spring back to life later, creating another episode of depression. If an individual is unable to work, improvement treatment works to get the employee not just back to work but working well.

The research strongly suggests that doing at least improvement-level work is likely to be cost-effective, regardless of who pays. Improvement-level work might look at personality traits, or it might look at contextual issues such as marital problems. Either way, gains may be greater and longer lasting. For individuals with personality problems, one may not even get necessity level improvement without also attending to some improvement-level issues.

Potentiality. The potentiality level picks up where improvement ends. Potentiality-oriented therapy works toward developing the individual's full potential. It focuses on overcoming the blocks all people must face before they can work and live as completely as possible. If client and therapist want to engage in such work, why would it be wrong? It is, however, understandable that third parties might not feel responsible for funding it.

Do We Charge Too Much?

Because therapy is intangible, one can easily become confused about its value. As therapists, we are more vulnerable to this problem than other people for two reasons. First, we make our living from therapy and thus are susceptible to imagining that we are overestimating its value for our own personal gain. The research suggests that, usually, the opposite is true. Second, we never took Business 101. Our lack of business skills prevents us from figuring out our true economic worth. Are people, including employers, better off economically after therapy than before? Do we give people their money's worth? The data say "Yes!" in a variety of ways.

Therapy and Medical Costs

There is an extensive body of research demonstrating that therapy reduces the cost of medical care by more than the cost of the therapy. This work includes but goes beyond the "cost-offset" research.

The cost-offset research examines the impact of giving psychotherapy to medically ill people on the cost of their medical care. Numerous studies demonstrate that the total cost of medical care for these people *actually declines,* even allowing for the cost of delivering the psychotherapy (Jones, 1979; Brody, 1980; Gonik et al., 1981; Kessler, Steinwachs, & Hankin, 1982; Schlesinger, Mumford, & Gene, 1983; Munford, Schlesinger, Glass, Patrick, & Cuerdon, 1984; Borus et al., 1985; Fielder & Wright, 1989; Massad, West, & Friedman, 1990; Cummings, Dorken, & Pallak, 1990). In other words, psychotherapy saves money in these cases. The Mumford (1984) article is a review of 58 other studies and concludes that overall medical utilization was reduced between 10% and 33% when mental health treatment was provided.

Research done with family physicians reveals that an astounding percentage of office visits are largely or entirely a result of psychological issues. To illustrate, Sheehan, Ballenger, and Jacobson (1980) found that 70% of people later diagnosed with panic disorder had seen 10 or more physicians before they were properly referred for mental health treatment. Other researchers (Brody, 1980; Orleans, Georges, Houpt, & Brudie, 1985; Kessler, Cleary, & Hankin, 1985) found that between 25% and 70% of office visits to primary-care physicians are basically psychological. Some visits are in response to psychosomatic symptoms, such as headaches, sleep disorders, and gastrointestinal disturbances. Many more are made by people who feel troubled and want to talk with someone who is knowledgeable. They pick their doctor.

According to the Summer 1995 issue of *Advance,* a publication of the Association for the Advancement of Psychology, 46% of psychotherapy in this country is given by primary-care physicians. Yet, 71% of such physicians said that they did not have time to address patients' concerns, and 32% said they did not have adequate training in mental health disorders ("Did You Know," 1995, p. 5).

The *Consumer Reports* study (1995) cited earlier indicates that people who consult family physicians for help with emotional problems are likely to get very little talk therapy but are highly likely to get medication (83%). Duration of therapy is usually under two months, and outcomes are not as good as for those who consult mental health professionals.

Several studies have found that people with untreated emotional problems are heavy users of medical services (Hankin, Kessler, Goldberg, Steinwachs, & Starfield, 1983; Borus et al., 1985; Cummings et al., 1990). This observation probably does not surprise you. People look for help where they can find it. We know that psychological and physical difficulties are intertwined in a systemic way. Contrary to traditional Western medical thought, each constantly affects the other. Coronary heart disease, high blood pressure, circulatory problems, migraine headaches, diabetes, and asthma are only a few of the physical disorders that have strong psychological components—in their causes, in their treatment, and in recovery. These diseases are among the most commonly diagnosed physical disorders.

For example, diabetes is known to create significant medical expenses. Treating diabetes successfully involves engaging the individual in a great deal of self-care. In other words, the individual must accept the diagnosis emotionally and then make significant behavioral changes. Emotional acceptance and behavior change are activities about which we are experts.

With regard to heart disease, research is growing that psychological and social factors are more powerful determinants of treatment outcome than is severity of heart damage. Those who are socially isolated, live alone, and lack a close confidant are more likely to die from a heart attack than others. One study (Berkman, Leo-Summers, & Horowitz, 1992) showed that people with no sources of support are three times more likely to die following a heart attack than people with two or more sources of support.

A study by Kiecolt-Glaser et al. (1993) provides evidence that marital conflict is associated with immunological breakdown.

Our society is beginning to understand mind/body integration. Popular works by Siegel (*Love, Medicine, and Miracles*), Chopra (*Ageless Body, Timeless Mind*), and Moyers (*Healing and the Mind*) articulate the profound impact that psychological and physical processes have upon each other. They identify how much people who have lived in our Western culture have lost by not appreciating these relationships.

Considering the body of research outlined in this chapter, one cannot help but conclude that our nation's medical bill would likely be substantially *lower* if the use of outpatient therapy constituted 6%–7% of our nation's health care bill rather than its current 3%–4%.

The Impact of Therapy on Business Costs

Psychological interventions offer great savings for business. The large body of evidence that supports this conclusion proceeds in three logical steps.

First, *emotional and substance abuse problems cost employers dearly*. Rice, Kellman, Miller, and Dunmeyer (1990) found that American business lost $77.2 billion in 1 year to these problems. Kamlet (1990) reported that $23 billion was spent on lost workdays. Kronson (1991) reported that substance abusers' productivity was reduced by 25%–33% in comparison to nonimpaired workers. Jansen (1986) estimates that *80%–90%* of industrial accidents are related to emotional or substance abuse problems.

Broadhead, Blazer, George, and Chiu (1991) found that depression increases disability days by 400% and absenteeism by 300%. The New York Business Group on Health surveyed 200 managers (reported by Rosen, 1991). Respondents to this survey reported that 13% of their employees experienced depression in the preceding 12 months. Of these:

- 36% had difficulty concentrating
- 35% had sleeping problems
- 27% had decreased energy
- 18% lost interest in their jobs

Clearly, these symptoms cost employers some tangible productivity and placed workers in danger of on-the-job accidents.

A study reported in the national press, undertaken by the Massachusetts Institute of Technology and The Analysis Group, found that depression generates $43.7 billion worth of costs for employers. This is approximately the same amount as that attributed to heart disease. Overall, depression costs employers $180 per employee per year (whether that employee is depressed or not!) ("Depression a Big Cost to Business," 1993).

Wells Fargo Bank of California (reported by Vaccaro, 1991) found out just how widespread emotional and substance abuse problems were among their employees. A well structured survey revealed that:

- 30%–35% reported several signs of depression
- 12%–15% reported enough signs of depression to qualify for a diagnosis of clinical depression
- 10% reported enough symptoms of anxiety to interfere with work
- 8%–10% reported a moderate to severe alcohol problem

Second, a large set of studies found that *treating the disorders that lead to these losses results in clinical improvement* (McClellan, Luborsky, O'Brien, Wood, & Druley, 1982; Steinbrueck, Maxwell, & Howard, 1983; Dobson, 1989; Harrison & Hoffman, 1989; Hayashida et al., 1989; Michelson & Marchione, 1991; Robinson, Berman, & Neimayer, 1990; Office of Scientific Information, 1992). In other words, our interventions are effective.

Third, and dearest to the corporate heart, several studies (Harrison & Hoffman, 1989; Spotlight: Managing Stress in the Workplace, 1991; McDonnell Douglas Corporation, 1990; Holder, Longabaugh, Miller, & Rubonis, 1991; Walker, 1991) found that *treatment programs actually produce savings.* These savings are achieved by improvements in productivity as well as by reductions in absenteeism, tardiness, dismissals, and disability claims. Interestingly, these financial improvements are not limited to employers. These same studies show that earned income of employees also rises. In other words, therapy helps those treated to earn more money, making therapy an investment, not a cost.

BellSouth, using Integrated Care (a program that *encouraged* outpatient therapy, developed in consultation with the American Psychological Association) reduced its mental health costs by $6 million over three years. These savings resulted from decreases in the use of *inpatient* mental health care.

The First National Bank of Chicago found that 14% of its health care costs were mental health based. To reduce those costs, they took the following three steps: (1) developed an employee assistance program (EAP)/health promotion program, (2) began a concurrent review of all psychiatric hospital admissions, and (3) changed the benefit plan to emphasize outpatient therapy. Over a 5-year period, while mental health improved, annual psychiatric hospital costs declined by $516,000 (59%).

Finally, Pelletier (1993) reviewed 47 studies of the cost-effectiveness of using behavioral interventions with employees to reduce health costs to employers. These studies looked at the cost-effectiveness of teaching healthy behaviors to employees. Programs included smoking cessation, stress management, and behaviors that reduce coronary heart disease. Forty-six of the 47 studies showed that the cost savings (usually far) exceeded the cost of the interventions.

Therapy Benefits and the Enhanced Financial Future of Children

Therapists help children to remove barriers to academic and personal success. Consider children seen in response to presenting problems of poor grades, based on anxiety, depression, attention-deficit/hyperactivity disorder (ADHD), disrupted families, poor parenting, and so forth. Left untreated, many such children continue a pattern of failure, acting out, and devastated self-esteem. With therapy, many of these children greatly enhance their capacity to achieve. (See Kazdin, 1993, for an excellent review of the status of research on the costs of childhood problems and the efficacy of providing interventions to children and adolescents.)

Therapy and the Savings in Crimes Not Committed

Finally, consider the savings in crimes not committed by those actor-outers that we help to find better ways to express themselves. According to literature of the Practice Directorate of the American Psychological Association, workplace violence cost American industry $4.2 billion in 1991. Employers who instituted a broad range of psychological interventions experienced a 10%–12% decrease in the number of attacks, harassment, and threats compared to employers who did not provide such interventions for their workforce (American Psychological Association Practice Directorate, 1995).

The August 1995 edition of the *Journal of Consulting and Clinical Psychology* presents a series of studies on the effectiveness of psychological interventions on antisocial behavior in children and adolescents. These articles demonstrate that we are developing useful tools for responding to these serious behavioral issues. Unhampered by issues of the medical model and third-party reimbursement, the authors were able to look at a range of interventions that respond both before and after the fact.

Despite these findings confirming our economic value, therapists continue to earn far less than our medical colleagues. According to a 1993 report from Reuters New Service, the average physician earns $180,000 a year. *Psychotherapy Finances,* in its 1995 survey of annual therapist income, found that the median incomes, by profession, were:

- Professional counselors $ 48,900
- Marriage and family therapists $ 53,300
- Social workers $ 59,000
- Psychologists $ 81,100
- Psychiatrists $116,000

OUR INTANGIBLE CLINICAL VALUE

Our self-esteem has been battered by our acceptance of managed care's accusations about our cost. The research just reviewed should show that we are not incompetent or unethical. The economic value received by clients far exceeds the economic cost. To complete the restoration of our self-esteem we also need to remember that the value of our services goes well beyond the cost issue. Beyond financial savings, we do a lot of good for people. That good has the most value of all. However, therapists tend to lose sight of it because we encounter it every day. Because it becomes commonplace to us, we forget how special it is to others.

> This was a family I had worked with before. They were genuinely nice people. This time they told me, "Our son is ill and may be dying. We need you to help us get through this time." Their son was 27, smart, good-looking, and wonderful with the children he taught.
>
> His death came after a number of months. One day, while he was still living, his parents were in my office. After about 20 minutes, I felt I was not being very helpful. It seemed as though we were just wandering around. I asked, "What could we do today that would be helpful?" They looked at me as if I had just said something particularly stupid. "We're doing it," they replied patiently.
>
> This was not a socially isolated family. They had both friends and extended family who loved them and cared about what was happening. However, nowhere in their lives did they find the particular kind of listening and freedom to talk that they were finding in my office. I was not doing anything that most of you would not have done. I just forgot how helpful it was. My fantasy probably ran to finding a way we could save their son. Fortunately, their reality testing was better than mine just then.

Consider the contributions we make to people's lives:

- We help people replace despair with hope.
- We help people replace incompetence with effective problem-solving skills.
- We help people replace terror with calm.

- We help people replace intractable conflict with understanding and cooperation.
- We help people replace misunderstanding with trust, and failure with success.

Who but us in this society is doing these things?

The clinical value of these contributions is every bit as high as the clinical value of treating ulcers, upper respiratory infections, cancer, and heart disease. Indeed, Wells, Stewart, and Hayes (1989) found depression to be as functionally disabling as several serious physical illnesses. They looked at 11,242 patients, 1,137 of whom were diagnosed with depression. People with hypertension, diabetes, arthritis, and gastrointestinal problems performed better on ratings of *physical functioning* than those diagnosed as depressed. All those with physical illnesses scored better on average than depressives in terms of social functioning. Only people with current heart problems did as poorly on physical functioning as people who were depressed.

One of the attendees at a seminar of ours in Boise, Idaho, was a young woman who had grown up in Hungary. She moved to the United States when she was 18 years old. When she came to our seminar, she had just finished her Ph.D. in clinical psychology. Part of her study took her back to her native country to examine their mental health system. She found that basically they did not have one. Someone asked her what Hungarians did about their mental health issues. "Alcohol," she responded. Everyone laughed. "And suicide," she added. The laughter died.

As this story illustrates, our society needs us to continue to offer our services in effective ways. If we do not, all of the clinical value we possess will be lost to ignorance. Consider another time in history when ignorance ruled. *Time* magazine ran a special edition on the coming new millennium and what we might expect. The writer described life in the year 999:

> Illness and disease remained in constant residence. Tuberculosis was endemic, and so were scabrous skin diseases of every kind: abscesses, cankers, scrofula, tumors, eczema, and erysipelas. In a throwback to biblical times, lepers constituted a class of pariahs living on the outskirts of villages and cities. Constant famine, rotten flour and vitamin deficiencies afflicted huge segments of society with blindness, goiter, paralysis and bone malformations that created hunchbacks and cripples. A man was lucky to survive to 30 and 50 was a ripe old age. Most women, many of them succumbing to the ravages of childbirth, lived less than 30 years. (Chau-Eoan, 1992)

The main reason for all this distress was ignorance of medical information that we take for granted today. We are now emerging from the Psychological Dark Ages, though the potential effect of managed care is to slow this emergence. Our society engages in behaviors, based on ignorance, that are as destructive as medical ignorance was in 999.

Violence is rampant in our society. Every day, some 14 or so children are murdered, mostly by other children. Too little is spent on education. (The average teacher in Switzerland earns $70,000 per year. Clearly, the Swiss value education more highly than our society does.) We encourage our children and teenagers to mature faster than normal developmental processes allow. This tendency distorts the developmental process, robbing our young people of skills they will need in adulthood. Families are hurried with too many duties and too little time for the nurturance they need to give and experience. Corporations know too little about the interaction of work and family stress and thus do not plan for it. Recently our local paper published the results of a poll that asked 11- to 14-year-olds, "When is it okay to rape someone?" Among the highly disturbing answers, 51% of the boys *and* 41% of the girls said it was okay if the boy has spent a lot of money on the girl. Our society *is still* in the Psychological Dark Ages.

On the hopeful side are changes we have seen recently in cultural attitudes toward drunk driving and cigarettes. Not long ago, people snickered about drunk driving. No one is laughing anymore. Social pressure and education are having beneficial effects on curbing smoking, as well.

Unlike the year 999, there are people around who have the needed knowledge to help move our society out of the Psychological Dark Ages. Many of those people are us. The question is whether we have the will to do the work. Will we make the changes in our self-definitions and our ways of practicing that will preserve and extend our true value? Or, believing the charges of managed care, will we become shadows of our former selves?

OUR FUTURE

The preeminent professions of the twentieth century have been medicine and electronics. Medicine keeps us alive, but it can provide neither meaning nor connectedness within that life. Electronics gives us great amounts of information but cannot determine what we do with it.

While many predict our imminent decline and demise, it seems clear that, if we take advantage of our opportunities, we therapists *can* be on the verge of becoming the preeminent professionals of the twenty-first century. We help people find meaning in their lives and make genuine connections with one another. These are some of the most powerful factors in determining quality of life. We help our society to become increasingly human.

SUMMARY

The charges managed care makes about the value of our services are simply wrong. Our services offer commanding value, both clinically and economically. We have a clear history of offering a variety of services that are well designed to meet the needs of those who come to see us. As we come to understand that value, our professional pride can be restored, and we can make better plans for our future than we would make if we continued to act as if managed care is on the right track. However, to make the best plans, we also need to know what mistakes we have made that have led us into our current dilemma. Chapter 3 outlines these mistakes. Understanding them means never having to make them again.

Chapter 3

The Business of Practice

Our profession is in trouble. To get out, we need to know where we went wrong, or we are likely to pick the wrong solutions. Managed care tells us that we have caused our own problems by keeping people in treatment too long and charging too much. *Our mistake is not in our practice patterns.* Research reviewed in the last chapter shows our practice patterns to be robustly effective and economically powerful. Becoming enslaved by the practice patterns required by managed care will only diminish the value of our work. Then we *will* be worth just what managed care is willing to pay.

The real core of our current problem is getting people to pay us what we are worth, for doing what we do, in the way we believe we should do it. This is a business problem, and it demands a business solution. Unfortunately, most of us did not get training in business. *Managed care is beating us with inferior services but superior business skills.*

The answer is to strengthen our business skills to gain control over our own fate, not to weaken our practice patterns. The first step is to give ourselves permission to learn these skills. To do this, we need a new attitude toward money.

MONEY AND THE HELPING PROFESSIONS

Money is at the heart of the crisis we face. It is such a highly emotional topic that many people, including many of us, have trouble discussing it. It is, in fact, the last taboo subject in America. Even in therapy, the place where people are supposed to be able to talk about anything, money often goes undiscussed. A client's financial history is far less likely to be discussed than his sexual history.

Our troubled feelings about money stem from our conflict between self-interest and wanting to help others. We would like to think of ourselves as selfless, and this part of our ego ideal makes it hard for us to recognize and accept our self-interests. Our feelings usually go unexamined in graduate training and supervision because our mentors have the same conflicted feelings. As a result, many of us find it hard to ask for the fee, have grave difficulties confronting missed payments, and avoid discussion of unacceptable payment plans.

Money and service delivery are inseparable. The money to access the resources of our services must come from somewhere, whether it be from fees, insurance, our own pockets, or taxes and grants that support agency work. By not facing the issue of money squarely, we have lost control of our ability to provide services the way we believe they should be provided. It may seem paradoxical, but only by balancing our selfless side with our need to take care of our self interests will we be able to offer ethical services of actual value to clients.

It is all right for us to want money. With money, we can take care of ourselves and our responsibilities. Without money, we become a burden on someone else. When we accept the idea that we have the right to earn a satisfying income, we acknowledge that we have the right to a place in the world and that our skills have value. We encourage our clients to believe these things about themselves, but we too easily forget to apply them to ourselves.

It is impossible, in the real world, to separate caring from practical issues. In fact, it is not good modeling to sacrifice our well-being to that of our clients when we are trying to teach them self care. The example we set is a far more powerful teaching tool than the words we say. The consulting room needs to be a place where everyone is considered valuable. Caring for clients and holding them appropriately responsible for services rendered are *not* incompatible.

How much money should we want? That is a personal issue, not a professional one. It is not up to our colleagues, our professional associations, or third parties to determine our income level. In private practice, we have to generate enough income to pay our office expenses and to support ourselves and our families in a manner that is commensurate with our skill level, educational level, and experience, and that does not leave us feeling angry, victimized, or burned out. That amount will obviously vary from person to person. If you earn too little or too much to suit *you,* the feelings of discomfort you experience as a result will ultimately interfere with your ability to do good work.

Not only do we need to earn money, *our clients need to pay us*. An underlying theme of most work with adults is helping them to behave in an increasingly adultlike way, an ongoing task for all of us. Although it often causes resentment, society expects adults to take care of themselves. Resentment of this expectation can be used as grist for the therapeutic mill. In the days when most therapy was paid for out of pocket, more was written about the therapeutic usefulness of discussions about money. If we are uncomfortable with our own feelings about getting paid, we are unlikely to make use of such therapeutic opportunities.

Adults expect to be responsible for what they use. When we require people to pay a reasonable fee, based on the true value of the service, we are treating them like adults. That is respectful and, in the end, builds self-esteem. While clients often do not begin therapy with a self-perception of adulthood, it does not seem like effective therapy to have structures within the therapeutic process that perpetuate immaturity. Overly helpful financial arrangements do just that.

Mr. H brought his 10-year-old son to see me in response to ADHD symptoms. These were being treated with medication, but it was not sufficient. Mr. H suspected that his son was also responding to his mother's inadequate visits (the parents were divorced). Mr. H was right. We spent 6 months of weekly therapy working through this boy's grief and damaged self-esteem. We spent a few more months in less frequent therapy.

Mr. H had a decent blue-collar job but was not rich, by any means. He was distressed that he could not himself give his son what he needed emotionally. He was proud to be able to pay for therapy. Doing so left his self-esteem intact, though it severely stretched the family budget. The budget eventually recovered. Had I rescued him from paying my full fee, it is not clear that his self-esteem would have recovered.

As helpers, we are vulnerable to boosting our own self-esteem by "helping" inappropriately. When we give in to this temptation, damage to our clients may result. Our helping inappropriately diminishes their sense of competence. It also robs them of a sense of equality in the therapy relationship. Therapy works best when conducted by equals, which is hard enough given that one person is usually not at his emotional best. However, if both client and therapist bring something of value to the relationship, something that is useful to the other, the foundation for a sense of personal equality is created. Clients need our expertise and our human caring. We need to make a living. Conducted on this basis, therapy is a win–win proposition.

Our conflicted feelings about money contributed to our vulnerabil-

---

BOX 3.1. Seven Facts About Money and Therapy

- Therapy is a professional transaction that involves the exchange of money for services. Money is part of what makes it a *professional* transaction.
- This exchange must meet the need of the therapist to make a living and the need of the client to receive quality service.
- We, not insurance companies, set our fees. Insurance companies are outsiders to this process. They have no power to mitigate our clients' debts to us.
- In paying therapy debts, money is a currency much superior to gratitude.
- Adults pay for what they use.
- Caring for clients and holding them responsible for what they owe are complimentary not incompatible.
- Relieving a client's obligation by absolving him or her of financial responsibility is disrespectful and disempowering, thus disruptive of the therapist–client relationship.

---

ity to the Siren song of third-party reimbursement. Because people could consult us with less personal financial sacrifice to themselves, we were able to avoid facing our feelings about the role of money in the helping professions. Insurance was so seductively convenient that we forgot that it is not a requisite part of the business transaction within therapy. In reality, if we provide services to clients, they owe us money for those services. If they want to use health insurance benefits to pay part of the fee, that is their decision. The nature of those benefits is a contract between clients and their employers. We are not a party to that contract. The contract between employer and employee has no necessary impact upon the client's obligation to the therapist. Yet, this fact often gets ignored. Even our professional associations seem ready to accept the idea that insurance is essential to therapy and that third-party payers are entitled to control what we do.

THE BUSINESS OF THERAPY: A BRIEF HISTORY

Paying attention to business has seemed ethically suspect in the past, but recent history teaches us that we need business skills to protect the ethics and value of what we do. The following is a short chronicle of how we got into our current predicament and why business skills—or the lack of them—*did* matter.

How We Got Involved with Third-Party Reimbursement

In the early days of our profession, therapy clients paid for services out of pocket. Of course, in those days, people paid for medical services out of pocket, too. Health insurance did not appear until the 1930s. Even then, it was only to protect people from the *catastrophic* expenses of hospital stays. Only later did plans such as Blue Shield appear, which paid for relatively small expenses such as visits to the doctor's office.

Through the 1950s, the relatively small number of therapists in private practice either saw mostly well-to-do clients or were satisfied with small incomes, often supplementing their incomes with jobs as university professors. Their work created a relatively small base of understanding within the lay public of the value therapy could offer. As that base gradually grew, opportunities for therapists grew because the value of therapy was becoming somewhat better known.

During the 1960s and 1970s, opportunities for therapists expanded dramatically with the creation of community mental health centers, funded through the Federal Community Mental Health Center Act. Jobs in these centers paid reasonably well and were wonderful opportunities to gain broad clinical experience. Demands for training increased. As more of us became trained, the interest in moving from the public sector to private practice also increased. However, private practice opportunities were limited because of the finite number of well-to-do people plus less well-to-do people who knew the value of therapy. Market saturation was easy to achieve. A way was needed to expand the market for mental health services.

At about the same time, in response to moderate growth of public interest in therapy, health insurance companies gradually began to offer mental health coverage. At first, following the pattern set by coverage for traditional medical services, only inpatient stays were covered. Then outpatient services gradually became covered, too. The cost of these add-ons was minimal because so few people used the services. The benefits were included as window dressing to help attract new corporate accounts.

Our profession had the business problem of needing to expand our market. The appearance of insurance reimbursement for mental health services was an answer to that problem—it just was not the *best* answer. Because we had little training in business skills, just as is true today, we did not recognize that there were alternative answers to this problem. Training in business would have taught us that there are two ways to expand the market for a product or service; either lower the price or increase the perception of the value. We chose to lower the out-of-pocket cost through health insurance, but unfortunately we realized too late that health insurance distorts the relationship between provider and client.

The decision to fight for entry into the third-party reimbursement system was a business decision. We will see that that decision could eventually have but one outcome—namely, to hand control of our services over to the third parties with the money.

In fairness to those of us on the scene in those days, it must be remembered that at that time it was considered unprofessional to advertise. Thus, we did not have the same options to educate people about our value that other business people had. However, in retrospect, we would have been better off had we mobilized our professional associations into undertaking effective public relations campaigns so that the public could get the information they needed about the ways we could be helpful. We would have fared even better had we had sufficient business skills to see that marketing can be integrated with professional ethics without contaminating them.

Pursuing health insurance reimbursement was a mistake also because of the relationship it put us in with respect to physicians and medicine. It seemed an opportunity to share a part of the prestigious position medicine then held in our society. We also believed that this prestige would help the public become more accepting of our services, enlarging our market even more. As we will see later, however, this relationship with medicine has had important drawbacks.

Initially only physicians were eligible for reimbursement for mental health services, and so battles were fought in state legislatures and in courts for "freedom of choice" legislation. For example, in the late 1970s, the Virginia Academy of Clinical Psychologists fought and won a landmark case against Blue Cross of Virginia that eventually went to the U.S. Supreme Court. The outcome of these battles was that health insurance companies were forced to recognize, first, psychologists and, later, other licensed therapists as reimbursable providers. This development solved the problem of expanding our market, but it created other problems.

Arthur Kovacs and George Albee (1975) tried to warn us. They noted how the medical model, which we must follow to get reimbursed under health insurance, would eventually contaminate how we think about and do therapy. We did not listen. The money was just too readily available.

As predicted, our way of practicing did become contaminated. We did not *want* that to happen, but it was an unavoidable consequence of the strategy we used to enlarge our market. It began with small, nearly unnoticeable steps, little compromises that did not seem to hurt anything. That approach made the next compromises easier, compromises we would not have made earlier. It went downhill from there. Consider the sequence of events.

In fighting for reimbursement, nonphysician therapists had to make the case, implicitly or explicitly, that we used the medical model, just like medical doctors. Health insurance, after all, pays for treatment of *medical illness*. Since this is the case, it is not too surprising that insurance companies expected us actually to follow the medical model in our work. Our feelings about doing so have been decidedly mixed.

During my seminars on "Building a Managed Care Free Practice," I ask participants, "What theoretical models do you use when you are actually in the consulting room with someone? Which ones best guide your decision making?" As you would expect from diverse groups of therapists, a sizable number of models are named: psychoanalytic, cognitive-behavioral, family systems, Ericksonian, humanistic–existential, gestalt, psychodrama, and many others. Thus far, not one therapist, out of hundreds who have been asked, has answered "the medical model." Not one! Yet the medical model, especially since the advent of managed care, has come to have a controlling impact on how we practice. Why? Clearly, it is not that we find the medical model to be intellectually compelling; otherwise, participants would mention it. The answer is simple. We followed the money.

Making use of denial, we at first failed to notice the impact the medical model had on how we conducted therapy. The reimbursement process was not that intrusive early on, at least for individual therapy. All we had to do was write down a diagnosis along with dates of treatment and identifying information.

We were told not to expect payment for marital and family therapy services. This upset us. We knew the value of family therapy but forgot that such services were certainly not born within the mental illness framework of medicine. If anything, they were born as *alternatives* to the medical model. In the amalgamation that we attempted to fashion, if a family wanted to access its insurance benefits, one of the family members had to be named as the "identified patient" and effectively take the blame for the family's troubles. Having an identified patient complicated the therapeutic process of understanding systemic issues in that it seemed to identify a candidate for scapegoating. It was next to impossible to integrate those two models elegantly. The pretzel was starting to twist.

Other intrusions followed, such as the refusal to cover services like biofeedback—still "experimental" after all these years—and intermittent refusal to cover certain diagnoses, such as conduct disorder or attention deficit disorder. More recently insurers have demanded to audit therapy records to be sure that they were kept according to insurance company rules and to find "errors in billing." When "errors" were found, tens of thousands of dollars were demanded from therapists in restitution. Decisions within the audit process were made by insurance company representatives, with little recourse available to the therapists involved.

Today, of course, the constraints that arise from relying on health insurance run the full gamut of reasons that we find to complain about managed care. Problems with length of treatment, external control of treatment, a limited range of theoretical models allowed, loss of privacy, and so on all result from using health insurance as our source of financing.

Had the full range of current constraints of third-party reimbursement existed 20 years ago, we probably would not have dreamed of participating. Because the constraints were imposed gradually, we have made increasing compromises in our practice patterns. We have complained, shouted in moral outrage, and despaired. Then we compromised. Our ignorance about business led us to believe there was no other way to get people to pay for our services.

The problems with the medical model go much deeper, and we will explore the implications in detail in the next chapter. The point here is that there is a fundamental law of business that we failed to recognize: *When you ask for other people's money, you unavoidably invite their control.* The day we accepted our first third-party check is the day we began to hand over control of therapy to outsiders.

Although we get enraged with the system, usually with good reason, we need to take a moment to look at the issue of control from the point of view of third-party payers. Imagine making a purchase but having no control over what you get. You go to the grocer for hamburger but must take and pay for steak. How long would you put up with that? Neither would insurance companies nor their clients, employers. If they were going to pay, they wanted to decide if they were buying steak or hamburger. It is no wonder that we are being controlled by third parties. We are taking their money.

Who do you believe should control the therapeutic process? If your answer is similar to that of the participants in our "Building a Managed Care Free Practice" seminars, you will say that you and your client should control the process. This belief, in combination with this basic law of money and control, dooms third-party reimbursement for therapy. No matter how third-party reimbursement is structured, those with the money will demand to control the process. The clear implication is that only the client's own money can be involved. If we do not acknowledge this law of money, our profession will continue to search for ways to "correct" the third-party reimbursement system, inviting history to repeat itself.

How We Lost Third-Party Reimbursement

Third-party reimbursement has had many undesirable consequences. But, for about 20 years, we did do well financially in that system. We got a lot of business, just as we hoped. This opportunity, imperfect though it was, is now fading, and we are upset by this turn of events. *What went wrong?* How did we lose the opportunity that we had developed? Once again, our ignorance about business is the culprit. In this case, we forgot to notice where our money was coming from and to nurture that source.

Recognizing the source of one's revenue stream is a business skill. Because we lacked that skill, when we tried to influence the system, we focused our attention on insurance companies. It *seemed* that was where our money came from. We got all caught up in their rules and their usual and customary rates (UCRs). We fought with them about what diagnoses and services were covered. It was a colossal waste of time and energy because the insurance companies were just carrying out the wishes of their clients, employers who bought the policies. Employers were the real decision makers. We never talked to them at all.

The issue of mental health costs turned really serious for business in the 1980s. Previously, mental health costs, even inpatient costs, were relatively minor items on the corporate balance sheet. The outpatient part of mental health was so tiny no one ever gave it *any* thought. Since it was a big deal to us, and because we fought with insurers so much, we imagined they were paying us a lot of attention. That was not true. Nobody cared.

Things began to change as mental health costs grew. In 1980, mental health accounted for 8% of the nation's health care bill. By 1990, that figure was 16%. This means that mental health costs increased at twice the rate of the medical consumer price index, which itself was absolutely out of control (Bak, Weiner, & Jackson, 1991). After a while, there was enough money on the table to draw attention. Money, like a loose football, tends to draw a crowd.

What caused this rampant escalation in costs? We saw in Chapter 2 that the outpatient component of the nation's health care bill continued to hover in the 3%–4% range during the 1980s. In other words, outpatient services did not contribute to this escalation. Inpatient care created this explosion in cost. Here is what happened.

In the 1970s, Diagnostic Related Groups (DRGs) were created in an attempt to control health care costs. These limited the length of stays for many conditions treated through general medical inpatient care. DRGs, however, were not applied to psychiatry. This meant that inpatient psychiatric facilities could keep people for as long as insurance coverage lasted. Coverage was usually a minimum of 28 days, while many policies paid for up to 365 days of care, with little or no outside review! As a result, for several years the profit potential for hospitals that was formerly available in general medical care could now be more readily found in psychiatric care.

As a consequence, the number of freestanding private psychiatric hospitals mushroomed. In addition, general hospitals raced to convert as many medical/surgical beds as possible to psychiatric beds. Between 1970 and 1986, the number of private psychiatric beds grew by 75%, from 7.2 to 12.6 per 100,000 population. Between 1986 and 1987 alone, the number of psychiatric hospital beds jumped 28%. This was not because our population suddenly became crazier. Admissions increased sufficiently to earn back the capital invested in these facilities. Admissions for adolescents and substance abusers in particular skyrocketed (Bak, Weiner, & Jackson, 1991).

The design of insurance benefits unintentionally contributed to the problem. Reimbursement patterns were far more generous for inpatient than outpatient mental health treatment. Probably the thinking was that inpatient care would place an undue financial burden on people, while most people could find a way to pay for outpatient treatment (remember that protection from catastrophe was the original purpose of health insurance).

With regard to psychiatric care, it became cheaper, in terms of out-of-pocket expenses, for parents of troubled adolescents to put them into the hospital for 30 days than to use outpatient services (Ackley, 1993). Of course, it cost insurers 500%–600% more, which eventually came out of employers' pockets.

Understandably, the business community became alarmed. Employers were particularly disenchanted with the "28-day cure," so called because many people seemed to be cured the day their insurance benefits ran out. Employers were also upset that many people, especially alcoholics, returned for several expensive stays without apparent lasting benefit.

This state of affairs tarnished the image of *all* mental health practitioners. Business did not differentiate between inpatient and outpatient practitioners because we had never explained those differences to them. It really is too bad we did not. There is abundant research that demonstrates that most people admitted to inpatient care do just as well with outpatient treatment. It just costs a lot less. (See Lowman, 1991, for a review of this literature.) We had a compelling story to tell.

By the late 1980s mental health costs were huge. Managed care companies saw a business opportunity that fit in with the long-range goal of gaining increasing control over the delivery of health care in general. If they could control the service delivery process, they could control their costs and profits. They established relationships with employers by focusing on issues of urgent concern to business. They worked hard to shape employers' buying preferences in the direction of giving managed care maximum control over service delivery. They developed plans to rein in what was now a mental health elephant. Business was receptive. Their attitude was: "We have to do something!" Outpatient therapists got caught in this much larger process.

By the time we saw what was happening, we were already in a deep hole. Managed care had delivered its message about who we are, what we do, and why we needed to be managed. Dislodging such a message, once it is effectively delivered, is hard to achieve. Because we had no relationship with employers, employers had no way of hearing how *we* would describe our work. It was *our* job to shape employers' perceptions of us, to let them know about our value. When we neglected to develop an identity with the business community, the main source of our income, managed care filled the void. And managed care officials created an image of us with their customers because it served their business goals to do so. It was not a flattering image.

Conclusion

A lack of business of practice skills led us to make decisions that in the long run have not served us well. We did not understand:

- The value of our services
- How to expand our market by educating people about the value of our services
- The role money plays in service delivery
- That third-party money meant third-party control
- The need to pay attention to our relationships with the sources of our income

A better understanding of business principles opens up wider options than we have otherwise. One of those options is the development of private pay services. It is a passive, dependent profession that leaves control of its fate to others. Let's not do that again. To control our own fate, we will have to add a reasonable set of business skills to our other skills.

BEYOND THIRD-PARTY REIMBURSEMENT: PRIVATE PAY PRACTICE

In a reasonable business contract, each person knows at the outset what his or her obligation will be. The advantage money has over all other currencies is that we know when our debts are paid. Clients can pay their bills in cash, not in gratitude or subservience. Taking payment in cash makes room for client empowerment.

The conventional wisdom, however, says that most people cannot afford to pay for therapy out of pocket. We have conditioned ourselves and our clients over the past 20 or more years to believe that third-party reimbursement is necessary to make therapy affordable. That is a perception based on business naiveté, not reality.

Let's look at some numbers. According to Pellitier (1993), $800 billion was spent on traditional health care services in 1992. An *additional $114 billion* was spent out of pocket on nontraditional (read unreimbursed) health care services. Some of these services, such as biofeedback, acupuncture, and so forth, might be considered mainstream. Other services are clearly not mainstream and may even fall in the same category as snake oil.

Why would people buy snake oil? Because, right or wrong, they perceive *value*. Because they perceive value, the issue of cost becomes secondary in their decision making. We have tended to believe that purchasing decisions are primarily a function of cost. Successful business people know that most buying decisions are made on the basis of value. The importance of cost varies inversely as the value of the good or service in question. The greater the perceived value, the less that cost enters into the decision making process. Contrary to our traditional understanding of how buying decisions are made, cost is secondary, except for products and services with low inherent value.

People spend their money on the basis of their priorities, which are established on the basis of their values. As they see new areas of value, people reorganize their spending priorities. There was a time, not long ago, when people did not make room in their budgets for cellular telephones, VCRs or computers. They do now. People will reorganize their priorities and choose to spend money on our services when they perceive value.

We convinced ourselves that only rich people could possibly afford to pay us out of pocket. What does this say about the value we saw in our work? People will not and should not believe in the value of therapy services if therapists do not. With apologies to the movie *Field of Dreams,* if you *value it,* they will *come.* If you do not value therapy enough to charge a rate that speaks to its value, they should not come.

Another factor for us to examine is what therapy costs and how that cost compares with other expenditures people choose to make. Earlier we noted that 90% of outpatient episodes are concluded within 25 visits or less. To find the total cost of the overwhelming majority of episodes, multiply your rate times 25. To make the math easy, assume a rate of $100 per session and a median number of sessions of 13. You can see that, under those circumstances, about half the people who see you will spend

$1300 or less, and most people who see you will spend under $2500. Some, of course, will spend much more. However, by the time they get to that point, they will know what they are getting for their money—and will value the therapy *accordingly*.

What are some things that people within most economic levels in our society spend money on? People find ways to pay for pets and their food and veterinarian bills, college tuition, automobiles, computers, home entertainment centers, VCRs, self-improvement courses (Dale Carnegie courses cost $995), legal fees, divorces, help with tax preparation, dental bills, and so on. Most people do not have insurance coverage to pay for dental braces; yet, many children ages 7 to 18 wear braces, despite a cost of about $3000 per mouth. Parents pay it because they perceive value. Some people who seem to have very little money manage to find enough for cigarettes, which now cost $15.14 per carton here in the tobacco state of Virginia. In a year, a person who smokes a carton of cigarettes per week will spend nearly $800. If both adults in the home smoke, the cost approaches $1600. Some people who are not rich find ways to get the money for radial keratotomy ($1200 per eye), liposuction ($2000 plus $1900 hospital fee), and face-lifts ($3500 plus $1900 hospital fee). (These figures are for Roanoke, Virginia, where the cost of living is relatively low; fees in other areas may be higher.) Recently a fertility clinic in St. Paul, Minnesota, reported that their fee is $14,000 per couple. Insurance does not pay. People pay for each and every one of these items *when* they perceive them to be higher on their list of priorities than competing items. Where does therapy fit in this list?

It certainly is easier for the rich to make such spending decisions. It is not just the rich, however, who make them. Most people within the broad middle class will obtain the products and services they desire if they perceive them as having sufficient value in their lives. For example, consumer columnist Jane Bryant Quinn (1996) reports that

> for all the talk about the high cost of higher education, middle class families are gritting their teeth and shelling out. . . . When selecting colleges, they're flocking to the higher cost schools. Instead of trading down as tuitions escalate, families have been trading up. . . . Young freshmen from families earning $30,000 to $100,000 are attending private colleges and universities in slightly higher proportions than they did 15 years ago, even though those schools charge considerably more than do public institutions.

Value determines where products and services fall in people's list of spending priorities. If we develop creative and honest ways to help people understand the value of our services, many more will choose to pay for them out of pocket. Fewer will say, "I can't afford it."

What about those who really can't afford it? Some therapists, in considering a private pay practice, have expressed reservations about leaving economically disadvantaged people behind. That is not something we want to do. Let's look at the problem. It has two parts. The first part has to do with determining how large a percentage of the population would not have realistic access to reasonable service. My experience thus far suggests that 80% or so of the population can make use of private pay services, especially with the payment plans to be discussed in Chapter 6. The second part of the problem has to do with finding answers for the remaining 20%.

The people at the low end of the economic scale need our services too. Finding a way to meet their needs has been a dilemma that has eluded a fully satisfactory solution by any system yet designed. Let's consider some alternatives.

One possibility revolves around health insurance reform. However, the economically disadvantaged will suffer the same ill effects from using insurance and buying into the medical model as everyone else. Further, great numbers of the economically needy do not even *have* insurance. Remember, to have insurance you either have to have a job with decent benefits or the money to pay the monthly premiums on your own.

Medicaid, which they may have instead, is not insurance, though it looks like it in some ways. It is an entitlement program much like Aid to Dependent Children and Food Stamps. At this point, Medicaid still allows choice of therapist but like an insurance program requires a psychiatric diagnosis and offers limited privacy and limited number of sessions. In addition, many Medicaid programs today are being shifted over to managed care/HMO-based models. Those programs will suffer from all the disadvantages managed care has to offer.

Another answer, one that therapists have used historically, is to provide some services pro bono. Professionals are expected to provide some services for the public good. There are many ways we may decide to meet this expectation, including offering free or highly discounted services.

Unfortunately, pro bono services alone cannot fill all the need. Private practitioners, unlike community agencies and free clinics, do not receive donations, grants, or subsidies to supplement their fee income. Therefore, clinicians in private practice cannot afford to see large numbers of people for much less than full fee and still pay their own bills without doing one of two things. Either they must, in effect, charge their full-fee clients for the needy person's therapy or work large amounts of overtime to recoup lost income. If full-fee clients are told that they are subsidizing other clients' therapy and choose to do so, there may not be a problem. This informing can be done by offering the same sliding scale fee to all clients, which allows everyone to make their own informed decisions. Private practitioners who see large numbers of clients for low fees, with no subsidies to offset these lowered fees, run the risk of burnout, either emotional, financial, or both. This is not good for anyone.

A third option involves community-based agencies, historically the first line of defense for providing therapy to the economically needy. However, in recent years, as some of their funding has dried up, many agencies have begun to move toward a private practice, insurance-dependent model of service.

Agencies and free clinics, because they *are* subsidized, are in a position to serve people of lesser means for a reduced fee. One means of providing pro bono services might be for therapists who wish to do so to donate some of their free time to such agencies, especially if funding for these agencies can once again come through taxes and charitable contributions. Unlike insurance money, which is earmarked for individuals, who, to get the money, must be branded with a diagnosis, subsidies are earmarked for the clinic. Individuals can pay a reduced fee out of pocket and still receive many of the benefits of private pay.

Of course, clinics are supported by third-party money, and the third parties, such as local governments or the United Way, will still want some outside control. However, that control can focus on overhead and clinic policy rather than individual treatment plans. There could be room for therapists to influence the philosophy, mission statement, and values of the clinic. They can make it their business to be involved with local government or the United Way to make sure that these values are understood up front and to assure continued adequate funding.

Some clients and practitioners may be willing to endure the disadvantages of clients using Medicaid or a reformed health insurance process, feeling that services obtained through these funding sources are "better than nothing." However, the agency model suggested here seems to have significant advantages in that clients can have access to services based on a wide variety of theoretical models, privacy can be better assured, and access to seasoned private practitioners can still exist to the extent to which those practitioners donate some of their time to these facilities, both in direct client contact and in supervision.

SUMMARY

We got in trouble because we lacked business skills, not therapy skills. Business skills are not inherently good or bad. How we use them can be good or bad. Let's use them for good. Before we can do so, we must learn them. While they are not simple to learn, they are not rocket science. Having read this chapter, you have already begun to learn them. We will return to business skills in more detail in Part II. For now, consider "Seven Points to Remember" (see Box 3.2).

BOX 3.2. Seven Points to Remember

1. We need a new attitude about money, one that fits both our ethics and how money works in the world.
2. Managed care beat us with inferior services but superior business skills.
3. We can expand our market by lowering our price or by teaching the public to value what we have to offer.
4. When we invite in someone else's money, we invite in their control.
5. The problems we face today result from depending on health insurance as our source of funding.
6. Private pay at full fee, with all its benefits, is a viable alternative to third-party reimbursement for at least 80% of the population.
7. Private pay at reduced fees within agencies or clinics subsidized by tax money, donations, and/or grants is a viable alternative to third-party reimbursement, including Medicaid, for the remaining 20% of the population.

Chapter 4

Conceptual Changes We Must Make

Our profession must move from a financially dependent position to one of proactive independence. This is significant change in terms of skill development, attitudes, and behavior. If the changes were not so far reaching, they would not be so hard, and we might have made them long ago.

As Stephen Covey writes in *The 7 Habits of Highly Effective People*, significant change can occur only from the inside out. If we are willing to make only superficial changes, we will be trying to build a new house on a partially rotten foundation. We will then wonder why our efforts failed. Developing adequate business of practice skills and attitudes, as discussed in Chapter 3, is one change that needs to be made. This chapter delineates three more changes necessary to make the transition: (1) letting go of the medical model, which defines human problems in terms of disease entities; (2) filling the resulting gap with an improved way of thinking about the work that we do; and (3) enhancing our psychological hardiness.

PROBLEMS WITH THE MEDICAL MODEL[1]

We rely on a variety of theoretical models to guide clinical decision making. But, because of how we get paid, the medical model has gained increasing control of how we practice. In fact, we may no longer be conscious of the medical model's full impact on how we practice. We need

---

[1] I hope that physician readers understand that my criticisms in this section are about a way of thinking, not physicians or medical skills, which can have high value.

to look carefully at the problems it brings so that we can let go of what is not helpful. Then we are free to use a viable alternative. Fortunately, that alternative exists. We have had it all along.

One thing we need to keep in mind is that the medical model is just a model, not reality itself. There are many maps of reality available. We should use the one that works best at any particular time. However, it is easy to slip into thinking of the medical model as reality because our culture accepts it as such. This is one way that it may have entered our thinking more than we realize.

Clients Must Be Ill

In order for people to access their health insurance benefits, they must be diagnosed as having an illness. Our work is then defined as treating *mental* illnesses. Declaring that someone has a mental illness has negative effects on the therapeutic process from the start.

Before managed care, these effects were less noticeable. Third parties demanded less of us, which meant that their kind of thinking intruded less into the consulting room. It was easier to deny that we were, to some degree, using a medical model approach.

Today, to gain reimbursement, it is no longer enough to list a diagnosis on the insurance form. We must document that illness in detail. To document illness, we must focus with the client on pathology. To do that, we must pay a great deal of attention to symptoms during our sessions, or we will not know how to fill out the forms or answer the reviewers' rather pointed questions. The more serious the symptoms, the more likely that we will win reimbursement, up to a point. If things look too chronic, managed care companies seem to use that as another reason to end treatment.

The more attention we pay to symptoms, the less time we can spend dealing with the underlying life issues that create these symptoms. Symptoms are almost always given as the presenting problem but are not the real problem. Medical model thinking, particularly as it has evolved under managed care, ignores this distinction. "Medical necessity" has come to involve getting rid of the symptoms and not much else.

Most symptoms can be best understood as an attempt, or the result of an attempt, to solve some problem in living. Usually this attempt is manifestly unsuccessful, or the person would not be sitting in our office. In addition, some people may be born with biological predispositions to have certain problems, such as difficulty in interpreting reality or having a body too drawn to alcohol. Such biological predispositions are likely to lead to problems in living. Our job is to help people to solve such problems, regardless of their source, in better ways than the person has found so far. The more time we spend focused on pathology, the less time that is left for the task of problem solving.

As *we* focus on pathology, we lead our clients to focus on pathology. The greater attention they pay to how "messed up" they are, the less they can focus on their internal resources for change and growth. This observation is consistent with Milton Erickson's thoughts about selective attention. None of us can focus on everything at the same time. As you are reading this page, you are unlikely to notice how your left foot feels inside your shoe—until you read these words and direct your attention to it. You *can* notice your foot. It was just not relevant before. We pay attention to what is relevant. If we, as experts, convince our clients that the truly relevant material is their pathology, they are likely to believe us. If we point them toward their strengths, they are more likely to find them. It is their strengths that will solve their problems.

Our natural talent is the facilitation of health and well-being. We, like the entire health care system, have become distracted by illness because that is where the money is (or was). Our new task is to develop a model that associates money with well-being.

Status Differential

The medical model creates an unnecessary and fallacious status differential between client and therapist. There are only two people in the room—one is supposed to be "sick" and one is supposed to be "well." An unspoken assumption is that only the sick person in the room has significant problems, while the well person handles life with the ease of James Bond. A myth is generated that being "well" means having no problems.

This dynamic is often especially visible during a family's first visit. If the family has already reached consensus as to who will be the identified patient, almost always a child or teen, a litany of complaints is presented by all but that child. The identified patient is likely to sit sullenly with eyes downcast. If you show this person any respect at all, there is usually a somewhat stunned initial response followed by what the rest of the family see as unusual openness. They think you are magic when you are really only respectful. If the child is less willing to play the sick role, he will argue energetically against the litany. Assuming someone in the family must be "it," he will identify all the "sick" behaviors of one or more parents. A game of tag ensues.

Identifying oneself as "sick" undermines a sense of general competence. When we do not feel reasonably competent, our discomfort can often reach a level that makes it hard for us to think clearly. This reaction hinders our ability to learn. By using the medical model, therapists hinder the learning that they are paid to facilitate.

The truth is, of course, that we are all struggling. We live in a highly demanding, fast-changing, stressful culture. None of us is born with all the skills we need. None of us has sufficiently broad life experiences that we are prepared for everything life may throw at us. Some people get thrown some real curve balls. Others who look "well" may not have been challenged yet.

Therapists are *not* better adjusted in every way than are others. A pretty wide range of adjustment is represented by the students in most training programs. Honest therapists will tell you that they often learn from their clients. Our special gift is our knowledge of the laws of human behavior, development, and change. But that gift has potential power only when mixed with genuine interest in and respect for the people sitting across the room.

All of us need to engage in lifelong learning. Different people need to learn about different things at different times. Someone currently labeled as schizophrenic may need to learn more about distinguishing between reality and nonreality. Someone currently labeled as depressed may need to learn more about the kinds of thinking that generate hopeful feelings. A company CEO may need to learn more about how to handle power in a way that draws the best performance from his people. A mother may need to learn how to access her patience in dealing with an impulsive, demanding child. A person who has used alcohol for anxiety control may need to learn alternative anxiety control methods.

Lifelong learning is a value. *The medical model defines the need to learn as a disease.* That *is* crazy!

Molly Layton (1995), in a wonderful article in *The Family Therapy Networker,* adds this:

> The capacity to "not know" yields an important difference between therapy and traditional medical treatment, with which therapy is too often and unfairly compared. Treatment in psychotherapy is different from the relationship between a knower (the doctor) and what is to be known (the condition of the patient). The condition is something there to be discovered, described and treated: pills counted out, hot compresses laid on, parts of the body cleaned, drained, swabbed or sutured, injected, cut away, splintered, bandaged. The body is there, pulsing, juicy, fleshy, responding, something to be acted upon, to be known. Whereas in psychotherapy (and nowadays in some more holistic medical treatments), clients are not there to be acted upon, they are not conditions to treat.
>
> In contrast to traditional medical practice, the energy in psychotherapy is fundamentally a co-creation between at least two people, and the therapist's own awareness is just as likely to want examining on the table as the client's. Such tolerance for self-awareness—mindfulness again—is a discipline cultivated by many schools of therapy. (p. 30)

The Medical Model, Personal Responsibility, and Empowerment

The medical model promotes a sense of personal helplessness about behavior: "I can't help it! I'm sick!" A recent cartoon suggesting the unofficial mantra of the '90s shows a tee shirt with the inscription "I'm a victim of _____" — just fill in your choice of mental disease. A popular variant is: "Maybe it's chemical."

Of course it is chemical. But it is other things too. We exist on many levels: biological, psychological, emotional, spiritual, social, behavioral, and chemical. What we do, think, or feel affects the chemicals within the synapses in the brain. In addition, the particular chemical mix within synapses may affect our mood and thus our behavior and thoughts as well.

The mistake is to reduce this multilevel interaction to simple linear terms instead of thinking systemically. A common error in Western thought is to confuse a physical correlate with the "cause." Then, as soon as we find a biological "cause," we impose a biological intervention rather than enabling people to learn more about their own strengths. Systems theory helps us to integrate all relevant elements, recognizing that each affects the other. Looking for the cause (i.e., biological vs. psychological) is often a waste of time. Looking for the most effective intervention is the key. In linear thinking, the identification of the initial cause too often depends on the discipline of the observer. The biologicalization of psychiatry creates linear rather than systemic thinking.

Consider how different the thinking of the medical model is from the theoretical models we favor when actually conducting therapy. Can you name one that does not encourage clients to take responsibility for their behavior? Each, in its own way, searches for ways to empower people so they can respond to the world more effectively and gain greater control over themselves. These models demand acceptance of personal responsibility regardless of how one came to be in a particular set of circumstances.

For example, someone who is raped should not be held responsible for having been raped. But, no matter how unfair the situation, that person must now take responsibility for gaining control of her or his response to being raped. Individuals must learn how to take control of their responses, or they will be forever imprisoned by the experience.

Some professionals have voiced concern that walking away from the medical model "leaves some people behind." They often cite schizophrenia and bipolar disorders as having powerful biological components. The argument being advanced here is not intended to disagree with that biological premise. The argument advanced here is that to think in terms of "diseases" tends to lead our thinking in less than helpful directions.

Eliminating the medical model does not eliminate consideration of biological, chemical, or genetic issues. For example, some people may be genetically determined to be more drawn to alcohol than others. Is this fair? It doesn't matter. These people must find the resources to respond emotionally, psychologically, and behaviorally to this challenge, or else they become its prisoner. To excuse people from this responsibility is an act of disempowerment. *Medical model thinking disarms people in ways from which many never recover.*

Similarly, some people may be born with a predisposition for extremely wide mood swings, leading to serious life problems. They too are responsible for finding ways to overcome this unfair disadvantage. Such methods may or may not include psychotropic medication. The argument advanced here does not disqualify chemical interventions as useful. I refer some of my own clients for psychotropic medication as well as continuing with talk therapy. This does not mean that we must think of such people as "sick." It just means that we are intervening by means of all the useful tools at our disposal.

A series of articles in the *American Psychologist* (Hunter, 1995; Corrigan, 1995; Heinssen, Levendusky, & Hunter, 1995) offers a competency-based strategy for working with the population currently called "the seriously mentally ill." The researchers report exciting outcomes. While they often continue to use the language of mental illness, because that is the common framework currently available, the methods the authors recommend show creativity and respect. As I read them, the models underlying their work do not require the use of a disease concept. Instead they focus on helping people effectively solve the problems in living created by what may or may not be biological predispositions and their responses to those predispositions.

It may help to recall the genesis of the medical model for emotional problems. In the early 1800s, people whom we now describe as schizophrenic were in some quarters thought to be possessed by the devil. In other words, they were considered to be evil. They were sometimes stoned to death because their bizarre behavior scared people. Calmer, more humane individuals, appalled by such cruel behavior, responded that these people were not evil — they were sick. These more humane observers chose a different cause on the linear continuum, one that seemed to eliminate blame. As a result, the luckier individuals were given what passed in those days for psychiatric care.

Human nature is not so different today. Weiner (1993) reported that people are quite willing to help those who have gotten into trouble through no fault of their own, such as having an illness that strikes out of the blue. People are less willing to help those perceived as having caused their own problems.

Suggesting to people that they are sick, helpless, or not responsible, an inherent component in the medical model, promotes failure and dependency. Too often people become their diagnosis: "I'm an alcoholic." "I'm a schizophrenic." In making such statements, people sum up their entire humanity in one word. No one word can capture any person fully. Too much of the person is literally lost as the person lives out the identity the diagnostic label offers.

Educator Darlene Stewart (1993), in another context, noted: "We must stop programming people for failure by lumping their weakest qualities together and assigning a label to it, such as learning disabled . . . mentally disturbed . . . trouble maker etc. Labels, more than describing limitations, become limitations in their own right. Labels become mental hooks on which people hang their thoughts about disability and failure."

What is needed is a model that empowers people by recognizing their responsibility for their own behavior without calling them "evil" or "sick," code words for "incompetent." Given that we all have problems, this model can apply to all of us all of the time. We already have many such models. They are the therapeutic theories we use in the office. We have done a poor job of helping our society to understand these models. In fact, as the medical model has insinuated itself into our thinking, we ourselves have had problems making the best use of these models.

The Destruction of Privacy

The medical model pathologizes our clients' secrets, secrets which no longer stay safely locked in our drawer. They now go to many places, some of which we may not realize.

Details about highly personal matters are routinely sent off to managed care companies and insurance companies. At the same time, managed care companies are going through great upheavals in ownership. So what? Suppose you are sending confidential material to the XYZ Managed Care Company, which has convinced you that it knows how to safeguard such information properly. What happens to that material when that company is purchased by ABC Managed Care, whose standards or practices might be radically different? When we release highly private information about people, we lose control of it. Large numbers of people may be able to gain access to that information, people for whom it is not intended. The computer age has brought us electronic medical records, sold as great tools for continuity of care. Perhaps they are. But I prefer to take my chances with privacy.

Reports of consultations are routinely sent by insurers to employers who provide health insurance benefits. An article in the May 18, 1994, *Wall Street Journal* demonstrates just how serious the situation is:

Many workers believe that their medical records are protected by doctor–patient confidentiality. But lawyers say this is more myth than reality. . . . the release forms that most workers sign in order to get insurance benefits automatically give employers access to medical records. . . . Employees who get reimbursed for visits to psychotherapists build up especially detailed records. . . . Companies generally don't start out with Orwellian intentions; they simply want to hold down expenses. But once the medical information is present, so are the temptations to tap it, for a variety of reasons that have nothing to do with keeping employees healthy, medical-benefits experts say. (p. 1)

Many insurance companies send information about their insureds to the Medical Information Bureau (MIB). The MIB collects medical and credit histories, making it accessible to its 700 member firms. According to *Kiplinger's Magazine* (Prodigy News Service, December 6, 1995), almost all companies who provide individual life, health, and disability policies that are sold in the United States and Canada belong to the MIB. Those firms use the information to determine whether to cover an applicant and, if so, how much to charge. *Kiplinger* says that about 5% of applications are adversely affected by MIB information. It was not until very recently that the Federal Trade Commission began requiring companies to tell consumers when information has adversely affected them.

Michael Freeny's article ("Do the Walls Have Ears?") in *The Family Therapy Networker* (1995) described one case:

Ultimately, Barbara's use of the "S" word (*suicide*), and the probable diagnosis of major depressive disorder it signifies, will become part of her computerized medical history, comprised of any claims for medical benefits she has made through a health plan, which is fed to the Medical Information Bureau (MIB) in Westwood, Massachusetts, a countrywide depository of medical information drawn from millions of clients insured by more than 700 member companies. . . . If Barbara seeks to join a new plan, or buy life insurance, this data will flash like a red-lighted morse code, blinking out the words "suicide risk." But Susan (Barbara's therapist) most likely does not know about the MIB, or even what exactly happens to the information about Barbara's suicidal thoughts that she taps out on her keyboard, no idea where it goes, who sees it. (pp. 38–39)

We had better learn what happens to the information we submit. We then need to provide an opportunity for fully informed consent when clients sign release forms for giving information to managed care. Otherwise, clients who are damaged by such release of information are likely to begin bringing suit against us.

Time magazine, in an article titled "Who's Looking at Your Files?" (Gorman, 1996), reports the following:

> U.S. Representative Nydia Velazquez, 43, knows how easy it is for medical secrets to find their way out of a doctor's files. When Velazquez was running for Congress in 1992 . . . someone got hold of hospital records detailing her 1991 suicide attempt and forwarded them by anonymous fax to the press. The *New York Post* broke the story, and Velazquez was forced to acknowledge publically something even her family did not know: She had tried to kill herself with sleeping pills and vodka. Despite the painful publicity, she won the election—and now she is suing the hospital for $10 million. (p. 60)

Reporter Christine Gorman noted in the same article, "More than a quarter of Americans responding to a 1993 Harris Poll said health information about them was improperly disclosed."

Finally, Ray Mount, a psychologist in Massachusetts who belongs to the Consortium for Psychotherapy, shared a number of vignettes about violations of privacy. Here is one:

> An abused woman, frightened by the prospect of yet another attack, attempted to get chemical Mace from her local police station. The police pulled her file, learned that she had been in psychotherapy, and required her to get a written report from her therapist before they would approve her request to carry Mace. The therapist, surprised to learn that the police had gotten the patient's medical record, investigated and found that it contained the information from the utilization review treatment forms which she had been dutifully filling out and sending to a managed care company.

In general, then, when a client comes for therapy, the only people privy to the client's personal problems are the therapist, the client, the client's employer, possibly the police, and potentially 700 insurance firms. The lesson here is that once the information is out, like feathers from a pillow, there is no retrieval.

As clients come to understand the risks they are taking with the details of their private lives, they are increasingly likely to hold back information. You may never realize they are doing so. You do know, however, the impact *that* will have on outcome. In fact, as therapy becomes less private, people are unlikely to come at all.

Health Care Reform

As the privacy issue illustrates, health care providers today are experiencing pressure to change how they practice—mostly for financial, not clinical, reasons. The majority seem to be succumbing to the pressure. To the extent that we hang onto the medical model, we are in danger of being dragged through health care reform, whether reform comes from the government or via the managed care industry. Right now, it looks like managed care is in control. If they mess up too badly, politics may demand that the government step in. Who knows what that will bring. It is hard to see a future for the broad therapeutic community in this burning house. Further, as noted earlier, managed care does not even want most of us.

Our Market

Finally, using the medical model *robs us of 90% of our potential clients*! The Rand Corporation did a wide-ranging set of studies on psychotherapy. Among the issues examined was the effect of the size of copayments on utilization of outpatient therapy (Manning, Wells, Duan, Newhouse, & Ware, 1984). In this study, the size of the copayment varied from 0% to 100%. Thus, when the copayment was 0%, therapy was free.

As predicted, more people sought therapy when the copayment was smaller. Yet, even when therapy was free, only 10% of the people would come. While estimates vary widely, those who use the medical model tell us that the percentage of people with diagnosable mental disorders is well in excess of 10%. When we eliminate the false distinction between well and sick, we can recognize that 100% of people have problems. So, why won't more people come to see us? What is the barrier?

One reason we have already discussed is our failure to educate the public about the value our services might have for them. But another problem is shame. People in our culture feel shamed if they see themselves as mentally sick. Fifty years or more of telling people that "mental illness is an illness just like any other illness" have not had much impact. One person looks at another, sees clear evidence of physical illness and says, in tones of caring and concern, "You're sick." The same person, seeing evidence of emotional difficulties or behaviors they do not endorse, says, in tones of disgust, "You're sick!"

Up to 90% of our population is unwilling to call themselves sick in this way. Perhaps their self-esteem is too intact. What should we do? Batter their self-esteem until they see what wretched wrecks they are? No. Our job is to present a more reasonable, less damaging model for them to use to access our services.

One hundred percent of people have problems. Thus far, we have largely been serving only 10% of them. If we continue to see ourselves as helpers of those willing to call themselves mentally ill, we have a serious market saturation problem. If we see ourselves as specialists in helping all people to learn and to change, our market is limitless.

Most of us complain about various aspects of the medical model. Yet, many of us insist on staying in a burning house. Why? John O'Neill, in his book *The Paradox of Success,* quotes Carl Jung's comment to people who enjoyed a recent, great success: "I hope it does not harm you too much." His point was that success can lead people to repeat behaviors that led to that success. Doing so makes sense until conditions change such that those behaviors no longer lead to success. Jung noted that many people continue to repeat old behaviors long after the benefits expire. People lose their willingness to learn, grow, and change—in other words, to take risks.

AN ALTERNATIVE

We already have numerous alternative models we can use instead of the medical model. They are the many well-developed theories of personality and schools of therapy that we actually use in working with clients. Psychoanalytic thought, family systems theory, strategic family therapy, cognitive-behavioral therapies, humanistic models, and many others are the models therapists report using when really with clients. We have valued them enough to use them in our offices and often to guide our personal lives. Yet, for the most part, we have not used them to help the public know what we have to offer. We have ignored valuable resources at our disposal.

While there are many models, reflecting the richness of the human experience, each model shares two common elements. Each identifies developmental and life issues (problems) that people face in living their lives, *and* each identifies useful skills that help people to deal with and master those problems. Because they all share these common elements, they can be subsumed under a general label, "the Problem-Solving/Skill-Building model."

These are not new terms, but I am using them in a slightly new way. Sometimes, when they are first exposed to this title, people think I am referring to psychoeducational activities. Others may think I am referring to a particular brand of counseling. Neither is the case. In this context, the Problem-Solving/Skill-Building model applies to all of our useful tools of therapy. Consider these examples.

When we genuinely listen, we help people to build the skill of listening to themselves. When we genuinely care about the people in the consulting room, we help them to develop their ability to care for themselves. When we empower people to be partners in the change endeavor, they develop the courage and faith to change.

We do not *cure* anxiety. We help anxious people learn self-soothing skills. We help them learn such skills in many ways, depending on the model we happen to favor and the needs of the particular client. Self-soothing can come from learning relaxation skills, or by resolving old hurts, or by learning new ways to relate to family, or by other methods we use. We teach people skills they can use to deal with anxiety, a natural experience in the living of life. Everyone with two brain cells to rub together will experience anxiety and must develop skills to manage that experience.

There is an old saying: "If you give a man a fish, you have given him a meal. If you teach a man to fish, you have taught him a skill he can use all his life." Similarly, if we only give someone a pill, we have relieved anxiety for the moment. If we teach people how to manage their anxiety through cognitive-behavioral modification, hypnotherapy, deep muscle relaxation or self-understanding/acceptance, these are skills they can use and reuse for an entire lifetime.

In like manner, we help depressed people develop more effective ways of thinking. We help histrionic people learn how to relate to others without undue drama. We help many deeply troubled people develop skills in self-awareness, self-understanding, and self-valuing. These are the skills that develop when someone listens carefully and caringly to what is said. People often need help in developing skills in the areas of trust, initiative, impulse control, facing reality, and problem solving. *Is that not what therapy is really all about?*

Rich Simon, editor of *The Family Therapy Networker,* asked me to write an article on my approach to developing the private pay market (Ackley, 1995). When I included a lot of material about the problems of the medical model and the advantages of the Problem-Solving/Skill-Building model, he responded, "Dana, you are preaching to the choir." This may be true. Most of you will probably find these comments consistent with your own beliefs. That is not the issue. The issue is what we have done with our beliefs.

Had we valued our beliefs as much as they merit (and had adequate business skills), we would never have been seduced by the medical model. So, it is not the goal of this section to necessarily give you new material. It is to remind you of what you already know and to encourage you to make better use of it. In the next few chapters, you will see how converting from the medical model to the Problem-Solving/Skill-Building model will offer many more constructive ways to relate to the public without having to compromise your theoretical positions.

Let's compare this model with the medical model.

Clients No Longer Must Be Ill

We no longer have to impose ideas of illness, nor focus unduly on weaknesses. We no longer have to imply that there are people who do not have problems—nor that that is something to be desired.

The Problem-Solving/Skill-Building model solves the blaming problem that the medical model tried but failed to deal with. People can have troubles without being sinful or helpless.

The Problem-Solving/Skill-Building model, in all its incarnations, offers people the self-perception of general competence while acknowledging the need for more competence in specific areas. Obviously, we must focus on the problems that bring people in the door to some extent, but time freed can now be spent on actually *solving* those problems rather than just *counting* them. This facilitates learning. It facilitates respect. It also makes it easier psychologically for people to come for services and stay long enough to get the full benefits of them. I can testify to this from more than 20 years of clinical experience.

A good number of the people who come to my office for the first time are reluctant to be there. My favorite illustration is an initial family session with a 13-year-old nominated by parents to be the "identified patient." As you know, people of this age have the primary developmental agenda of "fitting in" with their peers. Getting dragged to "a shrink" is not consistent with that goal. During their first session, most 13-year-olds sit sullenly while their parents describe, in gruesome detail, the difficulties that *finally* led to the ignominy of their showing up in my office.

During this process, I make use of opportunities to make contact with the adolescent. Then, somewhere in this interview, I say to him or her, "When I came to greet you in the waiting room, I could tell instantly that you are a person with problems." The usual response is for their head to jerk up, for them to glare at me, and ask, "What do you mean?!"—secretly fearful that I have seen something they have worked hard to hide. Even their parents look at me with some apprehension. My answer is, "As soon as I saw you, I could tell you were breathing. That means you are alive and that means you have problems." This usually wins a laugh from the teenager, and from the parents too. I go on to point out that I have problems, their parents have problems (this always gets a smile), my secretaries have problems, my family has problems, and so on. They are only too happy to agree. With very few exceptions, we can then really get down to business.

But aren't some people, you know, different? You may be able to think of people who *appear* to be generally incompetent, or sick, or disabled—call it what you will. Milton Erickson might respond that those people have come to focus on what they lack and, in so doing, invite us to focus on the same areas. Think of the people who came to your office who *appeared* incompetent to everybody (but you). As you began to help them struggle with the issues in their lives, you found evidence of strengths and possibilities that everyone, including these clients, may have overlooked. When they left your office, perhaps soon, perhaps years later, they no longer had that appearance.

Daniel Goleman's wonderful book, *Emotional Intelligence* (1995), gives us a natural language we could use in the Problem-Solving/Skill-Building model. Rather than talking about illness, we could talk about how our services help people enhance or strengthen their emotional intelligence. Who among us could not stand to have increased emotional intelligence? One advantage of this form of intelligence is that our quota is not limited at birth but can grow throughout our lives. As it grows, our success in life grows as well. What we currently call therapy, when it is successful, leaves clients with greater emotional intelligence.

Personal Responsibility

Therapy done with the Problem-Solving/Skill-Building model in mind begins with the question, "What can this person and I do together that will enhance this person's control over himself (or herself)?" Cognitive behavioral therapists focus on helping the person discover more useful ways of thinking. They do not do the thinking for the person. They offer the client empowering ways to think. Psychodynamic therapists work with self-understanding. They do not believe that therapist understanding will do the job. They hold clients responsible for developing their own understanding that they can take out of the office. Family therapists help families come to understand the interplay of family dynamics so that they can use that understanding to make changes.

All of these approaches hold the individual responsible for change. Change can only occur within a context of personal responsibility. People who avoid personal resonsibility cut themselves off from their own resources that can be used to better their situation.

Privacy

If we are not in the third-party reimbursement system, there is no need for outsiders to have access to our records. We are not asking for their money. They have no legitimate interest in our work.

To be sure, this does not free us from keeping good records. Reasons for having good records exist and will continue to exist, including helping us to plan and conduct our work, assisting successor therapists in the event of our death or disability, and protecting us in the event of malpractice actions. But the reasons will no longer include keeping insurance companies happy.

Health Care Reform

If we do not use the medical model, and we do not seek third-party reimbursement, we do not have to identify ourselves as "health care providers." Our professionalism has never been dependent upon being a part of health care. Managed care, and the impending disaster it is creating for health care, will be irrelevant to our practices.

This situation does not mean that our work does not influence health. We know that it does. It also does not prevent us from providing services to medical patients for whom gaining psychological skills will facilitate physical healing. It just does not have to be done from a mental illness perspective.

Our Market

A few decades ago, the railroad industry went through a severe shake-up. Many railroads that had been famously successful went out of business. Others thrived. What made the difference? Was it capital? The routes they owned? The quality of their equipment? Perhaps those factors played a role. The major difference, however, was self-perception. Those railroad companies that saw themselves in the railroad business got into trouble. Those who saw themselves in the transportation business did well. By broadening their self-definition, they found opportunities that previously were hidden.

We too have a choice. We can see ourselves in the mental illness business or in the Problem-Solving/Skill-Building business. The latter term allows us to continue working with everyone we have worked with so far, and opens up our availability to the other 90% of the population as well. In addition, as you will see, there are unlimited additional ways we will be able to provide services to people that have been hidden by a mental illness mind-set. We will be able to tailor our services around problems and concepts that regular people can understand, not mysterious disease processes they then wait for us to cure. This also makes it easier for people to make use of our services for the traditional needs. They become true partners with us.

Arthur Kovacs (1993), a strong voice in arguing against our engulfment in the medical model, presents his alternative to the medical model in terms of the "Life-Span Developmental Theory." This model holds that when people go through life transitions, the potential for trouble always exists. Examples of such transitions are divorces, children leaving home, people getting married, retirement, etc. People often benefit from consultations around these experiences.

You will find that there is an unending range of possibilities, many of which will be examined in later chapters. You will learn how to harness your own imagination to develop exciting opportunities that will serve you and your clients well.

WHY PEOPLE WILL FORGO INSURANCE

In March 1993, I attended the American Psychological Association's (APA) Leadership Training Conference. At that time, President Clinton's health care reform process appeared to be a done deal. Only the details were in question. Bryant Welch, Ph.D., then Executive Director of APA's Practice Directorate, presented us with a picture of what private practice would be. He ruined our day. The mood in that room full of 300 or more psychologists, most in private practice, was nearly utter despair.

As I listened, the attractiveness of walking away from the health care arena grew. "Let's just operate outside this ridiculous system!" was my attitude. After Welch's talk, I had the chance to discuss my idea with him. He looked at me with tired eyes and replied: "Dana, why would people pay out of pocket for something their insurance will pay for?" Dejected, head down, I walked away, mumbling, "They wouldn't."

He was right. People will not pay out of pocket for what insurance will cover. But what Welch and I both forgot is that insurance coverage for what really gives our services *value* is rapidly disappearing. This is a critical change. It drastically affects the answer to the question I posed, because *people make buying decisions on the basis of value, not cost.* They will pay out of pocket for services that are of demonstrably higher value than the services insurance now covers. There are four factors that make private pay therapy far more valuable than insurance funded therapy. With them, we are worth our hire.

Four Factors That Create Higher Value

Customized Attention

Leaders of the managed care movement tell us repeatedly that our profession is becoming industrialized and that it should be. They argue that shifting from a cottage industry to an assembly-line approach is just the inevitable course of business in America. Further, they seem to argue that our profession now knows enough about people to reduce problems to formulas with stock solutions. They are wrong on two counts. First, this is an incomplete vision of how American business operates. Second, we do *not* know enough to reduce human struggles to stock formulas. Hopefully, we will never delude ourselves into believing that is possible.

We already have enough pressure in our society to think of people in mechanistic terms. Individualized therapy offers relief from that pressure by recognizing individual worth and value. This cannot be accomplished via therapy formulas. Instead the hard work of individual listening and genuine responses from an interested therapist is required. David Elkind's landmark work, *The Hurried Child* (1981), while written about children, reminds us that everyone has an individual developmental pace. One person's developmental pace cannot be forced into someone else's formula without doing insidious damage.

Second, it is true that many aspects of manufacturing and business have become mechanized. McDonald's and J. C. Penney have done extremely well. However, there is still plenty of room for specialty clothing stores and restaurants that offer fine, customer-focused dining. Furthermore, successful large businesses are learning today that individualized customer service is critical for ongoing success.

Managed care really only wants a narrow range of the market. If they want that symptom- and illness-based, rigidly short-term kind of work, let them have it. The niche we want to occupy is based on quality, not price; and on strength, not illness.

If we are not careful, we will wind up trapped in a mind-set that permits us to think only as managed care wants us to. Our training institutions will focus only on teaching short-term therapy. The heart of our quality will be ripped away. We won't know how to get it back. The public, rightfully, will avoid us. Those who do not may conclude, "I failed therapy." They will not realize that therapy failed them.

An assembly-line approach cannot help but have a negative impact on therapy because of the factors that separate good from bad therapy. These factors include careful listening and individual attention. Our services can be responsive to the broad range of needs and wants clients have. Following Steenbarger's (1994) findings, we can offer brief therapy to those who have well-defined presenting problems, only want symptom change, are willing to do their homework, and already have strong interpersonal skills, just as we always have. We can offer other kinds of services to people who have other goals and needs.

Eliminating the Shame and Expanding the Market

High-quality service will help us to retain access to individuals already open to seeing a therapist. However, like any business, we need to create new markets. In our case, this means enlarging the percentage of people interested in seeing us beyond that 10% base identified by the Rand study. Since 100% of people struggle with significant issues in living, the sky really is the limit. If the first step in developing a successful private practice is maintaining quality, the second is normalization of the process of using our services.

We talked about changing our mind-set. We must also now communicate that different mind-set to help the public change its mind about us. Rather than using the language of medicine and managed care, we can use language that speaks to the real concerns people have. People will find this language much more inviting. Let's speak of stress, of negotiating life's changes, of problems in living, of learning new skills, of emotional intelligence. Not only is this language more inviting, people can understand it. And it does not make them feel crazy!

Real Privacy

A third important value of private pay is privacy. In fact, I am finding this to be the most powerful factor in my clients' choices to forego insurance payments. We know that people have enough trouble telling *us* their personal stories, much less the growing list of people who have access to our files. The impact of loss of privacy on the therapeutic process is still unknown, but it is likely to be high. As problems with privacy inherent in managed care come to the attention of the public, fewer secrets will get told in therapy. In fact, fewer people will show up at all.

Eliminating the Effects of Psychiatric Diagnosis

With private pay therapy there is no need for people to carry a psychiatric diagnosis. The positive impact of this factor on therapeutic process has already been discussed, with regard to both shame and personal empowerment.

Psychiatric diagnoses are coming back to haunt people in a variety of ways. Financially, many people have found that using health insurance benefits for therapy has actually cost them far more money than the cost of therapy. After making claims, many find that their health insurance premiums go up and stay up. I recently heard about a situation in which a woman diagnosed as depressed 15 years previously was charged higher rates due to that diagnosis. Life and disability insurance applications have been denied to people. Military applications and security clearances have been held up. Employment issues may arise, especially given the issues raised by the *Wall Street Journal* article on privacy cited earlier. With loss of privacy, the chances for these effects are ever higher.

With private pay, present and future employers, colleges, insurance companies, and HMOs do not have access to information about our clients. Our clients control that information and decide how it is used.

Those people in a position to make decisions that will affect our clients' lives will not even know our clients *were* our clients. The information will be private unless the client chooses to share it.

In summary, insurance no longer covers high-quality private psychotherapy. If people want it, they will now have to pay for it out of pocket. The value of private pay services is that they are individually tailored, nonshameful, more private, and more effective. If people want to pay less—that is, use their managed care benefits—they will get less.

If we do a good job communicating what we do, differentiating it for the public from services covered by insurance, people will see the value. When they see the value, they will buy our services. My own feeling is that, if I cannot sell my services on their merits, then I need to find something else to do for a living.

PSYCHOLOGICAL HARDINESS

There is one last internal change to discuss. We are in a crisis. Every crisis is a time of great danger and great opportunity. Will we succumb to the danger or seize the opportunity within this crisis? Seizing the opportunity will require us to be psychologically hardy.

Maddi and Kobasa (1984) did a landmark study on ways that people can respond to stress effectively. They did a 7-year study of middle- to high-level executives at Illinois Bell. These executives not only were going through the normal stress inherent in such jobs but also were fearful about the unpredictable effects of deregulation that occurred with the breakup of AT&T, the parent company. The intensity of change and disruption was enormous, similar to the enormity of what we face. Pelletier (1993), in discussing this research, notes that actuaries can predict that 20% of people experiencing this kind of distress will become seriously ill and that 5% to 7% will die.

The researchers wondered why some executives got sick and died while others seemed to thrive. Physical health histories did not give the answer. For example, a history of coronary heart disease did not push a person into the group likely to get sick.

What differentiated those who got ill from those who stayed well were psychological attitudes. Researchers found that three attitudes made the difference between illness and health, sometimes between death and life. They are similar to the attitudes that seem to help people recover from serious and life-threatening physical illness. They can be called the "three C's."

1. *Seeing challenge instead of threat.* Those executives who felt threatened by the changes they faced had trouble. They primarily experienced anxiety without much relief. It is understandable how that would wear down one's physical resources.

Those who did well said something like this to themselves: "Boy, this looks tough. But I have faced tough situations before, and I can do this, too." They recalled the various challenges of their lives and the successful ways they had handled them. Those memories gave them some relief from anxiety and confidence for the future.

2. *Making a commitment instead of practicing denial.* Those executives who denied the reality/size/extent of the problems got sick. As therapists, we have all seen denial at work and what happens when denial dissolves as reality overwhelms defenses. The emotional torrent can be devastating and sometimes engulfs the person's physical resources.

Those executives who made a commitment to change did well. Rather than use denial, they allowed themselves to view the reality of the situation consciously. Their commitment to change had two components. One commitment was to the self. It was a commitment to make a change in order to take care of one's own needs. Those who really did well, however, also made a commitment to something beyond themselves. They committed themselves to change for their family, or their church, or their company, or something else that was larger than just themselves.

3. *Taking control instead of lapsing into helplessness.* Those executives who experienced themselves as helpless got into trouble. In their perception, the external factors were in full control of life, while the executive's abilities were nothing. It was as if they allowed themselves to go through white-water rapids without even trying to avoid the rocks.

Those executives who determined that they would take control of the change process did well. They recognized that they could not control all the external factors that confronted them. They could, however, make certain that they controlled their own reactions to these factors in such a way that they had a good outcome. They did *not* say, "I will *try* to help myself." They *did* say, "I *will without question* make something good come from this."

We face an upheaval every bit as upsetting as the one these executives faced. Like them, we face losing our self-esteem and our livelihood. We can expect that 20% of us will get sick, and some of us will die. Psychological hardiness is a way of selecting which group to join.

You might *want* to engage in psychologically hardy attitudes and behaviors but feel you are not sure which things you actually need to do to ensure a good outcome. The rest of this book is designed to help you know what actions you can take. But the specific behaviors matter far less than the attitudes. The attitudes will lead to actions, and the actions will lead you directly or indirectly to where you want to go.

It is actually more important to move than to be sure you are moving in the right direction. A marvelous story illustrates the point. Some years ago, a military unit was lost in the Alps. They stumbled around for a while but clearly did not know where to go. The snow and cold were beginning to take their toll. Suddenly one of the men pulled a forgotten map from his pocket. Spirits rose! A path was identified. The men saved themselves. Only afterward did they take a really close look at the map. It was a map of the Pyrenees, not the Alps!

We don't always know where we are going when we start something. We don't have to. The most important thing is to find a way to develop an empowered mind-set. As people with advanced degrees, all of us clearly have faced serious challenges in our lives and met them successfully, even if just in terms of getting in, and then out, of graduate training. Consider further other challenges you have faced: developmental issues, difficult therapy situations, personal problems. Recall how you have met them successfully. Leave the failures alone for now, unless you learned valuable lessons you have since used successfully.

Make a commitment to yourself to change. Develop an appropriate amount of self-interest because successful change will not happen without it. However, you are not just helping yourself. You are also helping your society by helping to make sure that what makes our services valuable will continue to be available to it.

Finally, take control of your own reactions. Change what you can change about yourself to create opportunities.

Warning: Even with psychological hardiness, significant change does not come easily, even to people who spend their lives helping *others* change. Sometimes we like to think that because we are experts in the laws of human behavior, we are above those laws. This, of course, is not true. Knowing the laws provides us insight, which is useful, but insight alone is insufficient for change.

When people face change, five kinds of barriers are normal. If we are to change ourselves, then we must find ways to overcome each of the barriers.

Five Natural Barriers to Change

1. *Loss.* When faced with change, the first thing people think about is what they will have to give up. All change involves loss. Many people get stuck here, staying focused on what they will lose, unwilling to do the mourning, the emotional part of letting go.

2. *Awkwardness.* People feel awkward when asked to change. They

have to learn new behaviors and new ways of thinking that, at first, do not feel as natural or as comfortable as old patterns. Basically, we are not sure what to do. One personal memory is of being in the seventh grade at my first dance. Talk about awkward! How vividly I remember how badly I wanted not to go.

3. *Can I?* People wonder if they have the resources to change. Having never done the new things, it is a reasonable question. We often see a client's resources even when he or she cannot. It can be frustrating to us when people fail to see their own strengths.

4. *Isolation.* People feel alone during change. The distance between us and others seems to grow. This is especially true if we are making a change most others are not making, that is, when we go against conventional wisdom. People then sometimes choose to rejoin the group, even if it is marching lemming-like off the nearest cliff.

5. *Starting point.* When beginning change, people must begin from where they are rather than where they wish they were. The gulf between these two states sometimes seems so large as to discourage action.

The Bridges to Change

Fortunately, there are bridges over each of these barriers to change. While each of you knows them from the change-facilitator's chair, you may find them hard to see when *you* are the person needing to change.

1. *It is important to note your losses.* In my seminars, we spend time doing just that. Doing so helps the group move to the next step. Spend a few minutes right now writing down in Box 4.1 what you believe you will be giving up if you let go of third-party reimbursement. Let yourself identify specifically what you are worried about losing.

**BOX 4.1. Losses Involved in Letting Go
of Third-Party Reimbursement**

1. _____

2. _____

3. _____

4. _____

5. _____

The process of this activity in the seminars is interesting. Participants usually begin by identifying such issues as safety, financial security, and being in the mainstream. It does not take them long, however, to actually begin to note their gains, even though I have asked them about losses. They begin talking about "losing" paperwork, external controls, and violations of privacy. Against my initial instructions, they talk about gaining freedom and control. Getting *through* the loss barrier seems to free them to identify their desired, and realistic, gains.

2. *You can endure awkwardness.* I not only got through those first dances but eventually learned to enjoy them. We encourage our clients to endure awkwardness all the time. We should set a good example.

If your experience with change is like mine in the past few years, you will run into anxiety barriers many times. You will have sleepless nights, periods of intense doubts, and seemingly terminal confusion. When our clients tell us about these experiences, we know them as signs of potential growth. We do not say: "This is too much. Go back to your old ways."

Avoidance is destructive. One must move *through* the anxiety barriers. Know that you can. It helps to remember the energy burst that awaits you on the other side of difficult change. The excitement of my new activities and perspective is spilling over into my clinical work. I believe I currently am doing some of the best therapy of my career.

As people gain *information,* awkwardness and anxiety diminish. That is why denial is such a poor defense. While denial can diminish anxiety in the (very) short run, it actually intensifies anxiety in the long run because it blocks us from gathering information about our problem and thinking about potential solutions. This book will help you gain the information you need to make useful change.

3. *You do have the resources to change.* This is true on two counts, the resources you bring to the situation and the strength and fundamental value of your profession.

Again, consider other challenges you have met in your life. If you are a licensed therapist, you got yourself through some form of advanced training. Not everyone gets *in* those programs, much less through them. You have been watched and tested and have endured the stresses related to such examinations. Have you ever gotten a job? Have you ever gotten married or begun a family? What moral crises have you weathered in the past? What difficult therapy situations have you handled? All of these situations have called on your internal resources.

Your professional resources are also strong. Understanding the laws of human behavior and development is a powerful tool that can be used in more ways than have yet been imagined. Others value that tool, and still others will value it as they come to understand it.

4. *We can fight a sense of loneliness by communicating with like-*

minded people. If you begin to make the changes outlined in this book, you will be going against conventional wisdom. "Everybody" knows that surviving as a therapist today means getting on every managed care panel available. "Everybody" hates it but "everybody" is doing it. Those "everybodys" may be threatened or even frightened by your different approach to solving our common problems. They may be so depressed themselves that they may feel hopeless about your chances for success. They may worry about you. Or, they may worry that you *will* succeed and leave them behind. To relieve their own anxiety, they may try to talk you out of your plans.

The power of conventional wisdom is such that you will be tempted to conform. The solution is to keep company with some like-minded people in order to maintain perspective. Consult together, compare notes, enter partnerships—do whatever it takes to help you keep in touch with your own vision of your future.

I have at least two essential partnerships. One is with my professional partner, Louis A. Perrott, Ph.D. We have done business on a handshake for 17 years and are each the richer for it. We have learned to pick each other's brain, catch each other's mistakes, and settle each other down. We have kept each other out of a lot of trouble and together built ideas neither of us would have developed alone.

My other partnership is with my wife, Peg. As I pondered the decision not to join managed care, she and I had an honest discussion about our potential financial ruin. She never flinched. There was no question but that we together, with our children, would control our own destiny. That emotional support sustains me as I continue to bridge those anxiety barriers. In addition, Peg has a wonderful gift of logic and insight. Her contributions to the model of a managed care free practice are integral to its coherence and success.

It cannot be stressed too much—find a buddy (or two)!

Don't just dismiss those "everybodys." Their questions may help you consider problems you had not yet come to. Their challenges will help you identify some of the issues that will need to be addressed. When I do my seminars on "Building a Managed Care Free Practice" I often get asked questions I have not yet considered. Those questions have helped me further identify areas to explore and to consider.

I would like to see us redefine our relationship with society. My hope is that, through this redefinition, we can remove the barriers we have allowed to stand between ourselves and our society. As we make the changes outlined in this book, we will be starting a kind of quiet revolution. The fullness of change will not happen overnight but do not despair. We and our clients will begin to prosper immediately. As we encourage each other and spread the word, other therapists and their clients will prosper as well.

Soon we will not be alone. In the meantime, we will have to keep each other company.

5. *You must start from where you are.* You can do this when you realize that *the seeds for your future are in your present.* Some of those seeds are the professional skills you have. Some are the person you are, with your own unique experiences that will serve you in your changing. Keep both in mind.

A woman from Manhattan told me during lunch at one of my seminars: "Before I was a therapist, I ran a restaurant. I always had an advertising budget. I never thought of having one as a therapist. Now I can see what a mistake that is." She had, for a time, forgotten wisdom she had gained outside of her professional training. Our discussion of the need for basic business skills helped her remember that there are many sources of wisdom.

You may not be, right now, where you wish you were. Wishing won't change that, but careful assessment and planning will.

We have a choice. Will we behave on the basis of what "everybody" tells us is our future, or will we actively create our own future? Said David Lloyd George: "Don't be afraid to take big steps. You can't cross a chasm in two small jumps."

Summary for Part I

I hope you are getting fired up. The *how to*'s follow in Parts II and III. To make the best use of them, remember the following points:

- Our traditional services and our traditional practice patterns are effective and offer great value.
- Our value can be maintained and enhanced by operating outside of the third-party reimbursement system.
- Our value can be maintained and enhanced by disentangling the medical model from our ways of thinking and emphasizing those therapy models that serve us well. These can be subsumed under a generalized model that we can call the Problem-Solving/Skill-Building model.
- The services we deliver are of greater value than those offered by managed care. People will choose to pay for them out of pocket, if they know they exist and know their advantages.
- We got into trouble because we lacked basic business skills. Learning those skills will lead us to be successful in making our services known and helping people choose to pay for them.

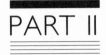

PART II

HOW TO BUILD A PRIVATE PAY THERAPY PRACTICE

In Part I, we looked at some of the conceptual issues that underpin our practices. This has not been an idle intellectual exercise. We did it in preparation for making changes. These changes will help you to design your practice so that its success will depend upon your own efforts, not the whims of others. In this section, we will take care of the practicalities.

In Chapter 5, we will consider issues important in making the transition from a third-party-dependent practice to one based on private pay. In Chapter 6 we will discuss services that can be offered to build your practice and methods your clients can use to pay for those services. In Chapter 7 you will develop a business plan for your practice. Finally, Chapter 8 will help you to learn how to market your services effectively.

Chapter 5

The Fundamental Strategy

Before beginning the process of changing your practice, it is necessary to create, in broad brush form, a vision of your future. This vision will help you to know how to apply the practical strategies that follow.

We are talking about change. Three states must be considered in making planned change: the present, the transition, and the future. Change theorist Richard Beckhard believes that the change process works best when we begin with our focus on the future. In other words, first we need to figure out where we want to go. The second step is identifying where we are. Only then can we adequately plan the transition.

Breaking Free of Managed Care is designed to outline the many possibilities for your future and to help you determine which of these paths will work best for you. The paths you eventually take will depend upon your vision of what you want. An exercise follows that asks you to give some focused thought to your vision. It's tempting to just keep reading, but I encourage you to stop here. Break the momentum. Find a pencil. Do the writing.

IMAGINING THE FUTURE: AN EXERCISE

Instructions This exercise (see Box 5.1.) has two steps. The first asks you to picture your practice as you would like to see it 2 to 3 years in the future. That picture may be fuzzy or vague. Generalities work fine for this exercise. Use whatever terms come to mind that feel meaningful to you. When you bought this book, perhaps some picture came to mind of what you hoped you would be able to do as a result of reading it. Call on that picture.

BOX 5.1. Developing Your Vision

STEP 1: THE FUTURE

List the 3–5 most important elements of your future practice. These may be services delivered, adjectives that describe what your practice *will be* (not what it won't be), client populations served, or any other terms you find yourself using to describe your vision. Tell what *you* want.

Important Elements

_____

_____

_____

_____

Main Funding Sources Desired *(rank them in order)*

_____ Indemnity insurance
_____ Managed care
_____ Private pay (neither you nor your client files for insurance)
_____ Institutional contracts
_____ Corporate consulting clients
_____ Your in-laws
_____ Other: _____

How much money would you like your practice to net (income minus expenses) three years from now? $_____   *(cont.)*

Step two is to describe your current practice. Doing so will help make sure that you have a clear vision of your beginning point.

In doing the exercise, don't worry about *how* you will make the transition. This book will provide you with strategies for getting from here to there. If you worry about the hows of the transition now, you will distort your vision of the future. When you have finished the book, then you can evaluate whether this vision of your future is achievable.

The purpose of this exercise is for you to create your own vision of your future practice, rather than simply accepting one imposed on you by others. As you focus on possibilities, you can gain a sense of direction

---

(continued from previous page)

STEP 2: WHERE I AM NOW

Now examine your current practice. What are the 3–5 elements that most clearly describe it? Again, these may be services, client populations, adjectives, or other terms that come to mind.

Important Elements

_____

_____

_____

_____

Main Funding Sources *(rank them in order)*

_____ Indemnity insurance
_____ Managed care
_____ Private pay (neither you nor client files for insurance)
_____ Institutional contracts
_____ Corporate consulting clients
_____ Your in-laws
_____ Other: _____

Current Business Structure

_____ Solo pactice
_____ Group practice partner
_____ Member of "group without walls"
_____ Employee of group practice
_____ Institutional employee
_____ Other: _____

How much money did your practice net last year? $ _____

---

and hope. Hope leads to action. This exercise serves to begin to create a map that can help guide that action. Since new terrain can get a bit confusing, having a map is important.

A SENSE OF URGENCY

It is unrealistic to imagine that you can close your old practice on a Friday and open a new booming practice on the next Monday. Instead, we are looking at a process of transition. Because your full transition will take some time, you need to consider getting started now. There is a *limited window of opportunity*. At some point in the next very few years, the old-style practice opportunities upon which most of us built our practices will be gone. At the same time, the doors to managed care "opportunities" will also be shut. Then you *will* be in a jam.

You can estimate how much time you have to make your transition by answering the following four questions which are outlined in Box 5.2.

1. *How much old-style indemnity insurance is left in your area?* Indemnity insurance is the kind we enjoyed the most — no panels, no reviews, just fill out the form and send it in. Most of us could find ways to live with indemnity insurance, though doing so nearly brought us to ruin. For now, indemnity insurance can provide some transition income as you go about preparing your market for alternative models. The more that is left in your area, the wider is your window of opportunity. Just don't get lulled into inaction. Be an ant, not a grasshopper.

2. *How willing are you to be on managed care panels temporarily or, like myself, work with clients as an out-of-panel provider?* While less desirable than using indemnity insurance, this option also can provide some transition income. Of course, the opportunities to join panels are decreasing rapidly. In most areas of the country, if you are not on panels now, your chances of being accepted are small. Frankly, I don't think you are missing much, but some therapists really count on panel membership for current income.

One potential danger of doing managed care work, at least in my experience, is that managed care/medical model thinking can insinuate itself into your frame of mind. The more that occurs, the more difficult it is to think in Problem-Solving/Skill-Building terms. When filling out OTRs and doing phone reviews, I found myself getting sucked back into the trance and fear of living with managed care. Others of you may be better at straddling the fence than I was. However, if you have been highly dependent upon membership on such panels, watch out. They are about to disappear.

3. *How much progress have integrated health care delivery systems made in establishing themselves in your community?* This is the next generation of managed care. The more such systems have come to dominate your market, the less that options 1 and 2, above, will be available, since these systems will replace both indemnity insurance and the current style of managed care, based on preferred provider panels. These systems may offer you employment opportunities, which, from my perspective, are unappealing. They will not offer you independent vendor contracts. To get one picture of this future, read "A Healthy Merger?" by Smolowe (1996).

BOX 5.2. Measuring Your Window of Opportunity

1. Indicate what percentage of your practice income in the past 12 months was derived from:
   a. Clients who used indemnity insurance   _____
   b. Clients who used managed care   _____
   c. Clients who used private pay   _____
   d. Other   _____

2. a. Are you willing to be on managed care panels for now? Yes   No
   b. What panels are you on and how many referrals did you get from each one?

   _____

   _____

   _____

   _____

   _____

   c. Are you willing to work "out of panel"?   Yes   No

3. What integrated health care delivery systems have set up shop in your area? What do you know about their progress in winning contracts with employers?

   _____

   _____

   _____

   _____

   _____

   _____

4. What financial reserves do you have to see you through a period of transition that may create a temporary reduction in income (hopefully followed by a period of recovery and improvement)?
   a. Savings _____
   b. Credit card limits _____
   c. Home equity _____
   d. Investment accounts _____
   e. Retirement accounts _____
   f. Other assets _____

---

4. *What financial resources can you draw upon during the transition?* During the 3 years prior to 1995, my practice income declined about 20%. The amount of income I lost was equal to what I would have lost had I taken the discounts demanded for belonging to provider panels. However, I was free of the hours of paperwork that managed care demands. I *invested* that time in developing the private pay model. My income is now recovering nicely.

In response to the income drop, my family did three things. We used some of our savings (that's what they are there for). We used some plastic—actually quite a bit. Finally, we cut back on some spending, though not a lot. We are not very good at that. Actually, that was not a mistake. While we were realistic about our financial situation, we never let ourselves feel poor. When people feel poor, they act poor. When they act poor, they do not experiment, and they do not make the investments of time and money required to move into new endeavors.

MY OWN TRANSITION

I started with a vision of what I wanted and assessed where I was at that time. How did I begin to go from here to there? My plan involved three components, but for now, let me tell you about the course of change in my clinical work, that is, the transition from a third-party-dependent practice to a private pay practice.

In response to an early practice slump, I had begun a newsletter (distributed to referral sources) in 1982, writing about clinical issues such as school phobia, helping children learn about work, peer pressure in adolescence, and other clinically relevant topics. I sent the newsletter to several hundred readers, including guidance counselors, principals, judges, pediatricians, family physicians, clergy, and others. It was a wonderful tool for generating referrals, literally saving my practice in those early years. To begin my transition, I sent an edition about the effects of managed care on the practice of outpatient therapy (see Box 5.3).

That issue, titled "Managed Care and Outpatient Therapy," described the kinds of changes that were happening and the way in which money drives managed care. Restrictions of service through 800 numbers, limited choice of providers, and utilization review were explained, along with the impact on the quality of the therapeutic relationship: "The net result is that whereas the provision of outpatient mental health services has been, until recently, a quality driven process, it is now rapidly becoming a cost driven process."

The newsletter also described our *apparent* dilemma: Cooperate or go out of business. I wrote that I was unwilling to take either choice. I

BOX 5.3. Newsletter to Referral Sources

Dear Reader:

Over the past 12 years, I have written this newsletter whenever I had fresh information to share. Past editions have dealt with problems such as ADHD, the effects of divorce on children, childhood depression, and so forth. This time the subject is not strictly clinical and yet has great clinical relevance: how managed care affects mental health treatment. It is an issue that many children, adolescents, and their parents are facing. Those who refer clients/patients to mental health professionals need this information to understand how services are being changed.

MANAGED CARE AND OUTPATIENT THERAPY

Health care reform is happening, whether Congress acts or not. Changes in health insurance design are multiplying. They affect what problems are covered, which providers are covered, and which clients qualify for reimbursement.

The changes increasingly pressure health care providers to change how they handle both the business aspects of practice and the services themselves. In mental health, the impact of managed care (MC) on the very nature of services is dramatic.

Changes may go unnoticed until people seek services. Many then discover that their coverage is only on paper. For example, one large employer in Virginia has a generous plan that offers 50 outpatient visits per year. However, the MC company hired to manage that benefit makes sure that few people ever actually have those visits. The reason is money.

THE MONEY PART

The purpose of MC is, of course, to save money. All forms of MC cut costs by limiting services. When unnecessary or wasteful services are restricted, the system has great appeal. But who decides what is wasteful?

Today, MC firms are given this task. Economics dominate the criteria used to decide which services are wasteful. Otherwise, competition puts the MC companies out of business.

It works like this: An MC firm offers to provide employees of the ABC Company mental health services for $X. It uses that money to pay providers and cover its other expenses. They assure the employer that they will provide "quality care."

Few employers are experts in mental health. They leave the defini-
(cont.)

(continued from previous page)

tion of quality to the MC company. The heavy burden of today's health care costs encourages employers to believe the MC company's assurances. Unfortunately, professionals have done a poor job of defining quality to employers. Thus, employers are not to blame for believing that what MC companies offer is quality care, even though it often is not.

Since it has many competitors, the MC company is motivated to bid as low as possible. The lower the winning bid, the more services must be restricted. If the MC company can administer and deliver the services for less than $X, it makes a profit. If it spends more than $X, it loses money.

RESTRICTIONS OF SERVICE

To save money, MC must deliver services for less than the employer was already spending while adding another layer of bureaucracy. To meet this goal MC typically restricts services in three ways: (1) MC creates obstacles to initial access, (2) MC limits choice of provider, and (3) MC limits treatment through "utilization review."

Initial Obstacles

Many people covered by an MC plan must first call an 800 number for "pre-authorization." This means that the caller must *justify* his/her need to the MC company. The MC representative, who may or may not be a mental health professional, will then decide if services will be allowed.

Those who have struggled to convince someone to seek services know how fragile that decision can be. An estimated 20% drop out rather than make this call. This reduces costs for the MC company. If the initial call is allowed to ring 8 times or more before being answered, another significant percentage give up.

Limited Choice of Providers

When the MC company does authorize initial visits, the caller is referred to someone on its provider panel. Practitioners selected for the panel usually have had to agree to use primarily short term treatment and have agreed to accept discounted fees. Reimbursement for clients who opt to see a therapist not on the panel is either sharply reduced or eliminated.

This means that clients are not free to select a therapist recommended by their doctor, minister, child's guidance counselor, or other tradi-

(cont.)

(continued from previous page)

tional source of useful information. Trust is one key to successful therapy. Referrals to a therapist from a trusted professional go a long way toward building trust between client and therapist. Referrals from MC companies are based on the economics of discounted fees and short term treatment, not trust.

Utilization Review

Utilization review is a process MC companies use to control how much care is given. They review each client's treatment to be sure it meets company guidelines.

If utilization review meant that professionals worked together to make the best possible treatment plan, this would be an excellent process. However, this is not what happens: (1) case reviewers usually have less training than the therapist; (2) reviewers have no direct contact with the client; and (3) MC companies have economic agendas that reviewers must serve.

For example, one large MC company demands that therapists average no more than six sessions per client. Reviewers must support those guidelines or lose their jobs.

When visits **are** authorized, most commonly only a few sessions are granted at any one time. When those are gone, a delay in treatment may be required while the bureaucratic process is repeated. Often no further visits are authorized, for reasons that mystify therapists.

Two side effects of this process impair the trust critical to the success of therapy. First, the stability of the therapeutic relationship is constantly in question. Second, the long tradition of therapy as a sanctuary of privacy is sacrificed.

Medical necessity: Increasingly, the phrase "medical necessity" is used as the benchmark for deciding when sessions are authorized. While this sounds reasonable, medical necessity is an MC term, not a medical one. MC defines medical necessity as helping someone get to a *basic* level of functioning. Anything more is considered beyond medical necessity and not the responsibility of the insurance carrier.

CLINICAL CONSEQUENCES

Such therapy focuses on symptoms while ignoring the underlying human issues that create them. It is like taking only enough antibiotics to

(cont.)

(continued from previous page)

diminish the symptoms of an infection. The infection comes back.

Thus, insurance coverage is now covering mostly short term therapy limited to problems that endanger life and basic welfare. It is a crisis oriented system.

People who rely on a crisis oriented system are in danger of having the same problems repeatedly, despite seeking professional help. This is because the real issues do not get needed attention. If this form of care becomes all that is offered, then people will believe they have failed therapy. They will not realize therapy has failed them.

The net result is this: whereas the provision of outpatient mental health services has been, until recently, a quality driven process, it is now rapidly becoming a cost driven process.

THE THERAPIST'S DILEMMA

MC troubles many therapists. Yet there is intense pressure to cooperate or be forced out of business. Cooperation means that providers must agree to offer primarily brief therapy. They must avoid asking for additional sessions "too often." Otherwise, their provider contract can be summarily canceled. The MC industry contends there are three times more therapists than are needed. So, does a therapist accede to the demands of the MC system or risk financial disaster?

Contrary to what the MC industry tells employers, outpatient therapists, as a group, have always been cost effective. I know because part of my response to the current changes was to seriously question my own style of practice. I wanted to know whether my practice pattern was wrong or if the changes demanded by MC were inappropriate. Therefore, I studied the research on mental health costs, outcomes, and cost effectiveness.

The MC industry has alleged that mental health costs are out of control. Research consistently shows that, in the outpatient area, this is not so. Outpatient costs have represented 3%–4% of the nation's health care bill annually since 1977.

The MC industry alleges that outpatient therapists keep people in treatment too long. The truth is that 90% of episodes of care are concluded by visit 25. A study of my own practice showed that 50% of my clients finish by the 13th visit.

Some people do need a year or two (or more) of therapy. In return,

(cont.)

(*continued from previous page*)

many of these people turn their lives around. Sometimes, in our "hurried child/hurried adult society," it is hard for people to be patient. With that mind set, long term therapy is valued less than it deserves.

MY OWN RESPONSE

Each therapist must make a decision about how to react to MC. Many therapists have signed up with one or more MC panels. They have worked out a relationship with MC that they feel they can live with.

One purpose of this letter is to tell you that I have made a different decision and will **not** join MC panels. Following MC treatment plans would be detrimental to my way of practicing therapy and therefore to my clients. I **will** go to reasonable lengths, in terms of paper work etc., to help clients to access their insurance benefits but will not allow benefits to control treatment.

Instead I will continue to deliver treatment that goes beyond crisis and symptoms. This means seeing people enough to get beyond the surface. It means realizing that symptoms are attempts to deal with a problem, not the problem itself. Adequately assessing the reason for symptoms and then dealing with them takes time. Part of good therapy is about taking enough time. I will continue to offer my clients that choice.

FINANCIAL CONSEQUENCES

Because of the long relationship I have with the broad professional community in the Valley, I wanted to take an opportunity to explain what I am doing and why. My approach may create complications in referring to me because of the *seeming* financial consequences. Let's look at them.

People are often misled by MC companies who say: "You cannot see Dr. So and So because she/he is not on our list." Or MC companies imply that treatment must end because reimbursement ends. Neither is true. People in America can still see who they choose to see for as long as they wish to see them.

Sadly, it will be increasingly true that more people, to get good care, will have to pay out of pocket. *This may not be as bad as it seems.* First, because of limits that exist even in traditional insurance plans, many

(*cont.*)

(continued from previous page)

clients have had only 40% *or less* of their charges reimbursed by insurance anyway.

Second, an unintended side effect of having had insurance reimbursement for mental health care is that many have come to believe they cannot afford treatment if insurance does not cover it. Even many mental health professionals, who should know better, have come to believe that myth.

In truth what *most people* can afford is a matter of priorities. Few people are wealthy enough to have everything they want. The rest of us make choices about what is important and what has long term value.

Money invested in timely, well-conducted therapy earns money in the long run. In the past 15 years, research has clearly shown that people who obtain appropriate outpatient therapy lower their general health costs **more** than the cost of therapy. People who have had successful therapy increase their earnings more than those who need but do not get it. The economic value of outpatient therapy far outstrips its cost.

When people have a clear picture of cost effectiveness, know that 90% of episodes of care last less than 25 visits, and can foresee the changes possible in quality of life, the priority of outpatient mental health care increases.

Certainly some people cannot afford therapy at all. For them the issue is economic survival. While most therapists offer pro bono services in one form or another, the reality is that the private sector cannot serve all of those individuals. Our society must make a concerted effort to adequately fund programs such as the Blue Ridge Community Services, Family Services, and The Family Place. However, many who now believe they cannot afford therapy will find it possible as they come to better understand the issues.

FORGOING INSURANCE

Today, many people who seek services have decided to forego their mental health insurance benefits entirely. They are finding advantages to this that include but go beyond quality of care.

First, privacy is maintained. MC, as you can see from its procedures, results in a sharp reduction in privacy. In an electronic age, increasing access to personal information exists as it floats around bureaucratic organizations. Disturbing reports of inappropriate access have been increasing.   *(cont.)*

(continued from previous page)

Second, access to care is on the clients' terms. They may see whomever they wish, whenever they wish, and for as long as they feel it is necessary. Treatment decisions are made jointly by clients and their therapists, not some third party in Minnesota. No paperwork comes through the personnel office of the clients' employers.

CONCLUSION

I appreciate the long relationship that we have enjoyed and look forward to working with you in the future. You may be assured that I will continue to provide the people you send to me the time and attention they need. Please call me (774-1927) with any questions or comments.

---

would continue to offer quality therapy and described the ways in which quality therapy had economic value. The newsletter concluded with a description of private pay therapy and its advantages. Referrals went up.

The next month I began giving new clients two handouts. The first described the pros and cons of using health insurance to pay for therapy. The pros can be described pretty briefly. The client pays less out of pocket for therapy. The advantages of private pay were then described: The client is free to choose whatever therapist he or she prefers, client and therapist control treatment, real privacy exists, and there is no need to run the risks inherent in carrying a psychiatric diagnosis. The second handout outlined payment plan options.

Historically, my practice had been about 10% private pay, that is, neither the client nor I filed for insurance benefits. (Do not make the mistake of defining private pay as occurring when the client does the insurance filing. That is still a third-party-dependent practice.) Within 2 months, my private pay income climbed to 40% of my therapy income. Within 8 months, that figure was 65%. Mixed with income from diversified services, which I began to offer in August, 1994, my practice income was 90% free of third-party payments within 17 months. My overall practice income recovered the 20% it had lost over the previous 3 years and continues to improve.

My own transition continues to be a work in progress. As part of my change, I have developed three components to my practice. Each of these three activities rests on the notion that my role is that of change agent rather than mental illness treater. This is consistent with my approach to therapy over the years, but my business methods are now much more consistent with my philosophy. The three components are (1) a self-pay therapy practice, (2) a diversification involving business consultation (to be discussed in Part III), and (3) diversification into helping therapists to change their practices—via this book, seminars, and private consultations.

Thus, progress has been rapid and encouraging. However, my situation may be different from yours. My practice and reputation were already well established. You may have a different starting point. That is why I am not suggesting that you just follow my exact steps. The goal of this book is to provide tools that will serve therapists with a wide variety of needs and starting points. That's why information and ideas have been gathered from a broad range of sources. My goal is to provide you a model, not a rigid recipe.

It is also interesting to note that my talking about these issues has led a great many therapists to call me. "I've had a third-party-free practice for years," some tell me. They just have not chosen to develop a model for the profession. The point here is that some therapists all over the country have found ways to operate outside third-party payments. You will not be alone.

THE OVERALL STRATEGY
FOR SHIFTING YOUR PRACTICE

If you are going to be in business, one of the first things you need to do is establish a market for your services. In the past, our strategy for doing this was to "hang out our shingles." Sometimes we supplemented this strategy with letters to referral sources, networking, and free speeches. We may even have developed a brochure that outlined our philosophy and described our professional services. Maybe we got some physicians and other referral sources to put some of our brochures in their waiting rooms. Finally, we put our names in the Yellow Pages. Then we waited in our offices for clients to appear.

In Part I we talked about expanding our market by educating the public, including the 90% who do not consider themselves "mentally ill," about the value our services might have for them. When people perceive that our services have something of value for them, those services become attractive. As our services move up people's list of priorities, they become more willing to see us and more willing to pay for our services with their own money.

If we are to expand our market in this way, then we need to change our marketing strategy. In general, there are three basic principles for us to follow in order to make our services *attractive* or of high priority to potential clients. You will find that these principles repeat themselves over and over again throughout the various applications that we will consider.

The three basic principles are:

1. Attractive services must speak to the *urgent concerns* of people before they will buy them. This means that we need to learn what feels urgent to people.
2. We must find effective ways to let people know that our services do speak to their urgent concerns. *People buy benefits, not features.* People care much more about the eventual outcome (benefit) than they do about the method you use (feature). A couple who want a happier marriage (benefit) do not care if you get them there via cognitive behavior modification or family systems thinking (feature). When we emphasize benefits in our communications with people, they can imagine why it would be worth their money and time to consult us.
3. We need to find ways to make it *easy* for people *to begin* the relationship with us. The more barriers we erect before someone can actually sit down to talk with us, the less likely it is that they will start. (Managed care knows this and uses it to help to *curtail* services, certainly not one of our goals.)

Applying these principals effectively is one of the business parts of practice. Let's outline the business skills that are required. The rest of this book will help you gain these skills.

RELEVANT BUSINESS OF PRACTICE SKILLS

To be competent in the business of practice, we must know:

- How to market
- How to do ethical selling (not an oxymoron)
- How to assess our competitors' strengths and weaknesses in comparison to our own
- How to price our services
- How to create a business plan

Some people are specialists in things like marketing and selling, having spent their entire lives learning about them, just as we have spent our whole careers learning about therapy. We do not have to become as knowledgeable as they are—we just have to be *good enough*.

Marketing

"Marketing" is a word that has long made many therapists uncomfortable. We developed the idea that telling about the value of our services was unprofessional because it could be done in manipulative ways. We equated marketing with telling slick lies. While marketing, like everything else, can be misused, that does not mean all marketing is bad.

The process of marketing is nothing more than a two-step process of education. The first step is learning about the needs and wants of potential clients. What is unethical about learning about what people might need or want from us? The alternative is deciding this for them from, as it were, ivory towers.

The second step in marketing is helping potential clients to learn about the value and availability of services we can provide. Without such knowledge, how would they ever know to call us? What is unethical about telling people about the possible benefits of our services, as long as we tell the truth? In fact, what are the ethics of having a service that could help someone and not letting him or her know? As we look at ways of marketing services to potential clients, I believe that your comfort level will increase, for two reasons: because you will see that marketing can be done in keeping with our ethics and because you will see that you can develop the skills to do it.

The goal of marketing is to develop interest in buying your services or products within targeted groups of people. If we can generate interest in our services, we need not worry about managed care companies delivering clients to us. Those companies sometimes say things like "We have access to 10,000 lives," as if lives could be totally under anyone's control!

Ethical Selling

If marketing makes us uncomfortable, the idea of selling drives us absolutely berserk! Before you indulge a bias, consider the following information.

Marketing is done to groups; selling is done one on one. It is personal. Images of fake smiles and pushing snake oil may come to mind. Like marketing, selling can be done unethically. It can also be done ethically. Millions of honest people make their living performing the needed service of selling products and services to people who want or need them. Like marketing, ethical selling is basically the same two-step education process—namely, learn about the client, let the client learn about you.

Consider how selling can be a service. When done ethically and honestly, it gives people an opportunity to learn about products or services they might really like to have. How can people find out if such products or services are right for them unless they can ask someone questions? Sometimes, that someone is you.

Now, consider this: every time you discuss therapy during a first interview, you are selling ethically, at least I hope you are. It is your job to present to the client the pros and cons of using your services. It is your job to help clients to understand how therapy can be useful, what benefits can reasonably be expected, what the alternatives are, and what costs can be expected, financial and otherwise.

Every time you talk with a potential referral source, you are selling. You are trying to convince the listeners that your services can be of value to people they might refer. Neither of these scenarios — "selling" to first-time clients or to referral sources — means that you are willing to cut the heart out of your mother to "make a buck." Purely and simply, you are educating individuals about something that you hold in high regard, and you hope they will, too.

Assessing the Competition

The goal of every business is to make money. I hope by now that this fact does not send shivers of shame up your spine. Like everyone else in life, you have a problem: You need to make money to support yourself and your family. You have chosen to solve that problem by having a therapy practice and doing things that really help people. If you do not make money in your practice, then you have not solved your support problem, and you have to find *something else* to do. So, in establishing a practice, you have to identify sources of income. *Others* are identifying the *same* sources of income as you. These are your competitors. As we have now seen, for example, managed care saw our former income stream and captured it. Because we did not fully realize what was happening, we did not figure out a way to protect our rightful share. Let's not let that happen again.

To keep history from repeating itself, you will need to learn how to notice who your competitors are. You will need to figure out what advantages you have and which ones your competitors have. You will need to figure out how to make the most of the advantages available to you.

This last statement does not mean that you must now become cut-throat, though some people do indeed compete in that manner. Most businesses compete in honorable ways, and you can too. You have always had competitors; many of them are your friends. Every private practitioner in your community is your competitor to one extent or another. Hopefully, you already have experience in competing with your friends without trying to push them into financial ruin so that you can have the biggest shop in town. We will look at how to assess your competitors so that you can make the most of your opportunities.

Setting Your Fees

Too often, we have allowed others to set our fees. We may have followed insurance companies' UCR rates or managed care rates. If we accepted these rates, then we had to build our costs around them. We did not consider the actual value of our services, as outlined in Chapter 2. We may not have considered all of our costs in doing business. Instead of setting an income goal for ourselves, we often just waited to see how much we made. All of this is passive–dependent behavior. It serves the need of leaving conflicted feelings about money unexplored, but it does not make for a well-run business. Therefore, we will look at the factors that are important in determining your fee structure. If you do not, you can easily price yourself right out of business. How does this serve your clients?

Making a Business Plan

Imagine this scene. Having put into practice all that you learn from *Breaking Free of Managed Care,* you find that your income has grown significantly. You have come to feel reasonably secure that you can continue to generate a good income. You and your spouse decide it is time to build that house that has been, until now, a dream. So you call a builder, and he says, "Great! I'll start tomorrow."

What's wrong with this picture? The builder has no plan! A house is a highly complex structure. If you do not create a clear plan before you start, three bad outcomes are nearly certain: (1) the outcome will be different from what you intended; (2) steps will be taken out of order, causing a lot of backtracking; and (3) eventual failure.

Building a business, which is what a successful private practice is, is also a complex task. It deserves careful planning. As you go through this book, you will get two opportunities to walk through the steps necessary to develop a solid plan for your practice. You will then use that plan to guide your decision making through moments of clarity as well as moments of utter confusion, much as you might use theory to guide yourself through the murkiest parts of psychotherapy.

The basic steps in making your business plan are:

- Determining what services you offer
- Identifying who you will offer these services to (who makes up your market)
- Determining how you will establish communications with your market (a marketing plan)
- Assessing your competition
- Setting financial goals

- Estimating your costs
- Setting fees that take into account both your financial goals and your costs

GETTING DOWN TO BUSINESS

The exercise at the beginning of this chapter asked you to create a vision of your future. I suspect that your vision included having a steady stream of clients calling for services. To achieve that part of your vision, you will need to overcome the barriers that keep people from calling you. What are they? They are the factors that make our services unattractive to potential clients.

In my seminars, I ask participants to identify those barriers. Here are some of the answers our peers have given: "Stigma." "People fear change." "People don't know anything about our skills." "People think we are crazy." "People are afraid we will think they are crazy." "People think they can't afford us." "People think therapy lasts forever." "People worry we will be like every critical authority in their lives." "People worry we will take control of their lives." "People think we are too permissive." "People are afraid we will hurt their marriages or families."

These reactions are the barriers we must overcome to create a private pay market. Given how little marketing we have done, it is not surprising people are relatively ignorant about us. In Chapter 4 we noted that, even when therapy is free, only 10% of people are willing to see us. In other words, as much as 90% of the population sees our services as either unattractive or without substantial value. To overcome these barriers, we will use the three basic strategies of (1) identifying urgent concerns, (2) speaking to benefits, and (3) making it easy for people to know us. We will use the basic business skills defined earlier to execute those strategies.

As the seminar participants usually note, one major reason people do not consult us is the shame typically associated with having a "mental illness" in our society. Authority figures often use shame in controlling behavior. It is not surprising that shame is effective in keeping people away from our doors. We have discussed how the Problem-Solving/Skill-Building model offers a path around shame. People do not have to see themselves as crazy, one-down, or incompetent to see us. Finding ways to let people know you operate within a different framework will help lower the shame barrier.

Another major barrier is that the majority of people cannot see how our services are relevant to them. We have not identified for them how we can be relevant. People buy services that respond to questions that they

have. They do not buy services because such services fit our pet ideas.
Nor do they buy services that are presented in our jargon. Thus, another
task is to find ways to communicate to the public, in their language, about
issues that matter to them. This is a shift in our marketing mind-set.

To demonstrate, imagine that you are sick and tired of wearing
glasses. Consider the following two ads from the yellow pages:

Ophthalmology   **Tired of wearing glasses?**
Eye Surgery   **We have alternatives!**
Board Certified   **Robert Jones, M.D.**
John D. Smith, M.D.   **Ophthalmologist**

Which ad is more likely to attract your call? Dr. Smith's ad is perfectly
proper and professional, but is he speaking to you? No, he is speaking
to himself. Dr. Smith's ad speaks to what he considers important, such
as being board certified. Do you know how an opthamologist becomes
board certified? I have asked hundreds of therapists with graduate degrees
of their own if they know. So far, about 10 have said yes. This suggests
that most people do not know and possibly even fewer care. Whether they
should care or not is irrelevant to marketing.

Board certification is an issue important to Dr. Smith and to the
faculty members of his training institution. However, Dr. Smith's former
professors are very unlikely to call him for services. Because board certification is important to him, he may imagine it is important to the public.
He has stayed inside his own head rather than putting himself in the public's mind to see what matters to the people he is trying to reach. He has
yet to consider seriously what potential new patients may feel is important to them. Perhaps, up to now, demand for services was high enough
that he did not have to know. Those days are ending.

Dr. Jones, on the other hand, *has* considered the people he wants
to attract. He has thought about what might lead someone to look in the
yellow pages for an opthalmologist. As a result, he offers a much more
attractive reason to begin a relationship than eye surgery. No one wants
eye surgery — ever! They may want the benefits of eye surgery but never
the surgery itself. Many people would like to be free of glasses. That has
value to them. Being free of glasses is a benefit. Eye surgery is a feature.
This example illustrates the "benefits versus features" principle that we
talked about earlier. People buy on the basis of the hoped-for end results
(benefits), not the means of getting there (features).

These ads also illustrate the importance of making it easy for someone to start a relationship with you. The more people have to commit
themselves up front, the less likely they are to make that initial contact
with you. Putting oneself at the mercy of a professional is difficult enough

in the first place. In his ad Dr. Smith implicitly says, "Unless you are willing to commit to my cutting on your eyes, don't bother to call me." Dr. Jones, on the other hand, implicitly says, "I'll be happy to see you about exploring alternatives. You do not have to commit to a thing before we meet."

Next, imagine that you go to see Dr. Jones to consider alternatives to glasses. Maybe you settle on contact lenses. Compared to radial keratotomy, this may not be a big moneymaker for Dr. Jones because it is a very limited service. However, you may give him repeat business for further eye exams and additional contact lenses. Furthermore, if you ever do develop a serious eye problem, whom are you most likely to call? You already know Dr. Jones—you have begun a relationship.

Now let's consider how our profession has approached its marketing. Look at the yellow pages ads in the therapist sections of your telephone directory. Those that go beyond name and address are making an attempt to draw business directly from the public. Yet most of those ads use our jargon, a foreign language to those people we wish to attract. Words like "psychotherapy," "anxiety disorders," "psychological evaluations," "clinical hypnosis," and "biofeedback" run rampant in our ads. *No one cares about this stuff but us!* When do you suppose was the last time someone woke up, turned to his wife, and said: "You know, honey, I think I'm going to run down and get a dose of biofeedback."

People are not beating down our doors looking for biofeedback or psychotherapy or any of those things. People are intensely interested, however, in the *effects* of those activities. It is the search for those effects that leads some people (namely, those desperate enough to do the translating themselves) to call us. If we change our marketing approach so that our communications focus on benefits and are written in everyday language, more people will see the connection between the effects they seek and the services we provide. This perception, in turn, should dramatically increase the chances that more people will call us. By speaking their language, we help to lower the barrier of ignorance based on language differences. By speaking about benefits, we lower the barrier of irrelevance.

Focusing on benefits is how products and services are sold. You are unlikely ever to want people to dig up your yard and lay drainpipes for $1500. However, if your basement leaks and a company says it can make it not leak, now you are interested. That's why their ads read: "End wet basements forever! Free estimate!" not "We will dig up your yard!" People don't buy a refrigerator because they want to spend $1,000 or more on a big, ugly appliance. They buy it to keep food cold. People buy benefits, not features.

Consider why you bought this book. You probably did not buy it because you wanted another 300-odd pieces of paper in your office, one of the features of the book. You wanted the benefit of learning how to have a managed care free practice.

Building a managed care free practice is a benefit that is of importance to you. My guess is that very few plumbers will buy this book. They will not even notice it. It is not relevant to their issues. It is relevant to yours, so you bought it. You were willing to make an investment because you thought the book had potential value to you. For me to sell you a book, I had to know what worries you have and speak to you about them in language you could understand.

But how much of an investment were you willing to make? You paid the cover price. Would you have paid double to get the value you seek? Triple? Quadruple? At some point, the answer changes from yes to no. Before you buy the book, its real value is undetermined. Whatever you spend is a risk. If this were my fourth book, and each of my previous books had been immensely helpful to you, then we would have an established relationship. In that case, you would probably have been willing to pay more than you would for my first book. We are only now beginning a relationship, so your willingness to risk is probably less.

Likewise, potential new clients will find it easier to make the choice to see us for a brief consultation the first time than to sign on for a year or more of therapy. In contrast to managed care, we may focus on brief consultations as an entry point, not as the end in itself. When we can offer worthwhile services oriented around brief initial consultations, we increase the likelihood that clients will become interested in building a relationship with us that goes beyond that initial contact.

We want to make it easy and attractive for people to start seeing us. After a relationship begins, people are willing to make more of a commitment. This attitude and approach seem appropriate. How many of you got married on the first date? Those who reply affirmatively, please call me to discuss boundary issues. Those who say they waited realize that clients must have a chance to get to know us over time before making a major commitment. This growing familiarity gives them a chance to become educated about what we really do and who we are. It helps them get past the cultural stereotypes that block so many people from calling on our services.

These examples are not intended to teach you about advertising per se. They are meant to illustrate the three key steps in marketing to the public. Remember, first you want to get inside the heads of your target audience to figure out what they perceive to be important. Second, you want to describe how your services respond to what is important to them in ways they can understand. Third, you want to find easy ways for people to begin a relationship with you. In some businesses these are called "entry-level services." Here, entry level is not a description of your experience level. Instead, it refers to entry into a new relationship. It is easier for people to decide to buy small services than larger ones. Keep that in mind as you develop your new strategies.

The Problem-Solving/Skill-Building model lends itself beautifully to implementing these marketing principles. When we begin thinking about problems rather than psychiatric diagnoses, we are taking giant steps toward talking about issues relevant to potential new clients. We are beginning to speak their language. They want to solve problems in their lives, and they use their own language to understand those problems. We do not want to create a barrier between them and us by requiring them to learn our language before calling us. Most people will not do it.

None of this changes the basic services we offer. We will still provide more extensive therapeutic services where appropriate, just as we always have. It is just more likely that people will test us with short consultations first. How we offer them, how we frame the invitation, will be different. The services themselves, however, have value and will be retained and, in fact, enhanced.

SUMMARY

In this chapter, we have identified the three basic building blocks of a successful business: knowing what people want from us, letting them know we have it, and making it easy for them to get it. These building blocks have been used by all kinds of successful businesses. We can see how these processes can help to overcome the barriers that may obstruct people from calling us. In Chapter 6, we will consider specific ways to put these concepts into practice.

Chapter 6

How to Learn from Your Market and Where That May Lead

In this chapter we will look at how you can determine the urgent concerns of people. Then we will look at the kinds of services that this knowledge might lead you to offer. We will also see that shifting to the Problem-Solving/Skill-Building model will help us speak about our services in terms of people's urgent concerns.

LEARNING YOUR MARKET

The first step in creating attractive, easily accessible services is to learn about the needs and interests of the people you want to serve. You need to know how your skills overlap with what is of interest to the public. How can you find out? You can do a market study. However, you may not know how, and you might be worried about the expense. It cost the Virginia Academy of Clinical Psychologists $22,000 to do its market study. Few of us want to spend that kind of money on a market study. Fortunately, we do not have to. There are at least three ways you can do a market study for free!

Free Market Study Method I

You bought this book because it spoke to an issue of yours. People buy books all the time because they speak to their relevant issues. Go to any bookstore, and you will see a wall of books dealing with issues of living. Some of these books have genuine value. Some do not. Whether they have real value or not is irrelevant to this exercise. When people buy them, they tell us what is on their mind. That is the relevant issue for us in assessing a market.

Consider these examples. *Men Are from Mars, Women Are from Venus,* by John Gray (1993), has been a runaway best seller. Whenever people buy this book, they are telling us that issues of heterosexual relations are both important to them and in need of some attention. As you peruse bookstore shelves, you will see what looks like 7,893,456 books on parenting. Whenever people buy one of those books, they are telling us about concerns they have in raising their children. They are not only concerned but also willing to spend money and at least consider changing their behavior. It is not hard to fathom why relationships and child rearing are subjects of urgent concern in the daily lives of many people. The idea of framing services in terms of emotional intelligence is supported by the tremendous amount of time Goleman's (1995) book spent on the best seller list.

One free way to do a market study, then, is to go to local bookstores and find out what books people are buying. Publishers have done much of the work for you because they only accept books to publish that they have reason to expect will sell. Your examination does not have to be done as precise science. The goal is just to get an idea of the kinds of books that are selling. Then notice which of the issues within these books are relevant to the issues that fall within your areas of expertise. Now you have some ideas and language that you can use in offering your services to your community.

Also, visit the magazine rack. Check our the types of articles that are being written for magazines targeted at specific audiences, especially those of interest to you: men, women, teens, executives, the health conscious, etc. Magazine publishers study their market to determine the issues of urgent concern to their readers. You can piggyback on their research.

Free Market Study Method 2

As professionals, we are accustomed to reading journals to gain useful professional information. Given our interest in the Problem-Solving/Skill-Building model, wouldn't it be nice if there were a journal that identified the problems that bedevil people's lives? Good news! There is! It comes out every day! It is the newspaper!

The newspaper is a daily collection of reports on problems that matter to regular people. If you use a marketing eye as you scan the headlines and read selected stories, you will notice issues that relate to your areas of expertise.

Suppose, for example, that you like to do work in the area of relaxation and anxiety management. You might then have noticed a story like the one in my local paper several months ago with the headline "Airline Courses Can Help You Take the Fear Out of Flying." The story reported that airline companies contract with therapists to help people get over flying phobias. This is in the mutual interest of airlines and people who want to fly. Maybe you could link up with the local offices of carriers in your area. Or perhaps you could make contact with travel agents who are also likely to run into this problem.

There are probably opportunities described in the paper every day. You may not have seen these opportunities before simply because you were not looking. Now that you are, you will find them. I am writing this on a Saturday morning. To test the process, I examined some of today's headlines. It took me 2 minutes to find a winner: "Bad Stew? Just Hide the Review." The story related how a college food director hid 4,000 copies of the student newspaper because an article in it panned his food— naturally, just in time for parents' weekend. Of course his act was immediately discovered. Now he not only had to deal with a bad review but also with the consequences of his poorly conceived reaction, as well. My guess, not knowing the man at all, is that he probably responded impulsively, making a bad decision under considerable pressure. Lots of people make bad decisions impulsively.

The point is that, upon encountering such a news story, a voice inside you might shout, "Eureka!" Perhaps you could offer services focused on "decision making under pressure." Decision making is a human issue that affects everyone. It is a skill building issue. We know a lot about decision making and about pressure. We work with people all the time on such issues. People do not have to be ashamed of themselves for wanting to improve decision-making skills. To make it attractive, be careful about the language you use in talking about it to the public. We *could* call the service something like "ego skill development therapy," which would prove to our peers how well we understand our theory of choice. However, our goal is to be inviting to the public, not to impress our peers.

This example came from picking up the newspaper that happened to be available today. Who knows what will be available tomorrow?

Free Market Study Method 3

Pick someone with whom you had an appointment this week—anyone. Now recall the life issues that led this person to contact you originally. These may or may not be the presenting problem. Write down these issues, but be careful about your language. Do not use any DSM terminology or other kinds of professional jargon. Jargon can obfuscate our meaning, especially to ourselves. Use language your mother would understand, unless your mother happens to be a therapist too. Whatever you write down is an issue of such urgent concern that it compelled that person to seek your services. You have now done a small-scale market study.

In our seminars, therapists have offered many excellent examples of this process. One woman told of a 10-year-old boy whose parents brought him to her because of "social isolation." This boy needed help in learning skills relating to making friends, which included changing some of the ways he thought about himself and about others. It also involved learning some behavioral controls. The *issue,* however, is a normal life issue. All children need to figure out how to make and keep friends. All parents worry when their children have difficulty with it.

The therapist who contributed this example could offer services to children in her community on the topic of "secrets of making and keeping friends." This phraseology would be a welcome switch from framing the services as appropriate mainly for "troubled children." Some children seen in response to this offer would likely want and need only a few sessions to achieve their goals. Others—whom we might once have branded as having some psychiatric disorder—may need to stay longer. You just made it easier, gentler, and safer for them to find you and get started by electing to use an inclusive approach to marketing.

A more extreme example was offered by another therapist. His client was a man arrested for the fourth time for exhibitionism. The therapeutic tasks included helping this man develop both impulse control and an alternative method for having a personally satisfying sexual life. While the solutions this man had developed prior to therapy were inappropriate, the underlying issues are not. Sexual satisfaction is an issue of concern to almost everyone.

Which attitude is more likely to make this person perceive your services (and whatever new learning is inherent within your services) as attractive—"You are a pervert!" or "You have not yet learned how to have a reasonably satisfying way to enjoy your sexuality"? Which attitude is more likely to win cooperation on therapeutic tasks?

Now think of it from a marketing perspective. One approach offers shame. The other normalizes the issue, though certainly not the behavior. Shame over sexual feelings is likely a powerful factor in the problem anyway. How does it enhance treatment outcome to increase the individual's sense of shame by calling him a pervert or giving him a diagnosis?

One more example. A therapist described a woman who had overdosed on alcohol at Christmastime. The five preceding Christmas holiday periods with her family of origin had also been disasters. The woman had difficulty controlling her use of alcohol, and she had equal difficulty handling her family's controlling behaviors. Death by drink seemed a more attractive option than another Christmas like the ones she knew firsthand.

What is the underlying issue? Well, we could call it alcoholism, but I have noticed that most people seem to resist accepting that label. We could say that the woman is having a major depression. The serious, nearly successful, suicide attempt, as well as her longtime low mood, could certainly support those labels. Neither of those, however, identifies the central life issue of greatest concern to her.

The underlying issue is control. The woman was allowing alcohol, her family, and her moods to run her life. Beneath all the symptomatic behavior, however, this woman was genuinely interested in learning how to run her own life. Who isn't? The therapist in this case suggested that he might relabel the services he offers as "running your own life when others want to do it." Remember that the suicide attempt came at Christmastime, a time this woman found her family to be especially controlling.

Now, go to your files. Take out the files of your 20 most recent new clients. Write down the issues that brought them to your office, in non-jargon language. What life problems are represented that are of such urgent concern that even the current barriers to seeking your services were overcome? What are the skills that need to be built or improved? The answer to that question will tell you something about the needs in your community. You will have also translated individual issues into language that might help you to communicate with others in your community who might have the same preoccupations and concerns.

The answer to the question of issues and skills will also tell you how your community currently views you. Are you happy with this collective perception? Are these the issues you want to be known for? If so, you need only to figure out additional ways to let the community know you. We will explore how to do so in Chapter 8. If not, you need to change how your community sees you.

What are the life issues that grab your interest? It is around those issues, the ones that turn you on and about which you are knowledgeable, that you will do your best work. These are the issues around which to build a practice. A participant in the seminar we held in Manhattan, Sarah Hardesty, Ph.D., offered a modification to our suggested exercise that seems apt. Rather than looking at the 20 most recent clients, in relation to the issues that brought them to her door, she looked at the 20 most recent clients whom she had enjoyed working with the most.

USING THE KNOWLEDGE

Once you have begun identifying issues of urgent concern to others, you need to translate that knowledge into services that address those concerns.

The most exciting part of doing seminars on "Building a Managed Care Free Practice" occurs when participants' imaginations start to percolate. As we begin the 20-client exercise in the third free market study approach, ideas always begin slowly. After the first new idea or two get expressed, the pace quickens dramatically. Suddenly ideas are expressed that have been cooking in someone's mind but were blocked by conventional wisdom and the rules of third-party reimbursement. As those restrictions are lifted, people begin outlining new ways that they can be helpful. One idea builds on another.

Since you are probably reading this alone rather than surrounded by a large group of people, you do not at this moment have the benefit of group synergy. Therefore, I have included some examples designed to stimulate your imagination, just as the group's energy and thoughts seem to stimulate those present. Some of these examples come from my practice group, some from the newspaper exercise, some from participants in our seminars, and some from a variety of other sources. The goal is not to give you an all-inclusive list but rather to fire your own creativity. Listening to hundreds of therapists generate ideas, I have learned that our possibilities are almost limitless.

Members of the Manassas Group have built their practices providing traditional therapy services, just like most of you. Over the years, some of the services provided have evolved to fit some aspects of the approach being outlined in this chapter. You may find that these services sound familiar to you in that you or your colleagues already provide them. These are traditional services, but the therapists have attempted to frame them as relevant to issues important in real life rather than framing them in terms important to third-party reimbursers. In so doing, the therapists involved have been filling a niche in the community and strengthening their practices. These services can reach their full potential as marketing methods are continually improved.

ADHD Clinic

In our community, as perhaps in yours, one might think from appearances that about 856% of children are diagnosed with attention-deficit/hyperactivity disorder (ADHD). In other words, professionals have taken a reasonable concept and have overapplied it. Some professionals appear to be diagnosing ADHD within a 15-minute office visit. Diagnosis often appears to rest on such criteria as whether the child takes the professional's office apart during the visit or how strident the parent or teacher is in complaining. Unlike most DSM terms, this one is popular right now among the general public. It relates to questions people actually have about their children and themselves, and because of that, using this term may help to interest parents in calling us.

Three of us—Louise Lampron, Ph.D., Kaye Longley, Ed.D., and I—
worried that many children hurriedly diagnosed with ADHD actually have
various emotional difficulties simultaneously expressed and hidden by outrageous behavior. Alternatively, a variety of family difficulties can lead
to disruptive behavior that is too often equated with ADHD. Finally, many
truly ADHD children come from dysfunctional families whose problems
are ignored in the rush to treat the child just for ADHD.

What is necessary is a careful workup that asks the question "What
best explains this child's problematical behavior?" rather than "Is this child
ADHD?" A series of individual and family interviews, done by one of the
two clinical child psychologists on our team, is the first step. We take a
detailed history, get to know the child, and get to know the family. Ques-
tionnaires completed by parents and teachers are included. Medical and
academic information is also acquired.

On the basis of this assessment, a decision is made jointly by parents
and professional as to whether a formal psychometric evaluation by Dr.
Longley, the school psychologist on our team, will be done. She has developed special interest and expertise in the assessment of ADHD. She
is also skilled in the assessment of learning disabilities, often a concomi-
tant issue for children with ADHD-like symptoms. Finally (and rarely),
if necessary, one of the clinical psychologists does a projective psychological evaluation.

The total fee for this evaluation runs between $800 and $1,000. (The
fee is higher if projectives are needed.) By the time we finish the evaluation, we have established a relationship with the parents and the whole
family. We have established our credibility. Parents often talk about how
they trust our opinions because those opinions have been carefully developed. The evaluation is an example of a service that managed care may
not pay for but that many parents want. It is a niche for us, and it is somewhere for parents to turn when they want the best and managed care is
just not good enough.

We are now in a position to deal not only with ADHD but with other
contributing issues, as well, if needed. Frequently, parents of difficult-to-
manage children need to learn some special parenting skills. Russell Barkley
(1990, 1995) has developed an excellent training program for parents of
ADHD children, which I have found useful for parents of a variety of
difficult-to-raise children. The program lasts between 6 and 10 sessions.
Moving through this program deepens my relationship with the parents.
As a result, we often move into traditional marital and individual therapeutic endeavors.

Let's go back to our use of the term ADHD, which I said was popular with the public right now and so would not pose a jargon problem
in terms of marketing. How does the use of this term fit with my beliefs

about the medical model? Recall that I am giving up the medical model, not the biopsychosocial model. Research on what is called ADHD, particularly by Barkley, is persuasive to me that there are some children who probably have a biological characteristic that promotes behavior that is troublesome to them, to their parents, to their teachers, and to their peers.

My concern comes when we label this condition a disorder. In my clinical experience, many children and their parents have been disempowered when the word "disorder" is attached to this condition or characteristic. ADHD becomes an excuse, not an explanation. As a result, when the families get to us, much clinical attention must be paid to reempowering both the child and the parent to cope with the cards that were dealt to them. In order to get to this point, however, they have to get into our offices. Because of the widespread attention to the term "ADHD," using that term in our marketing may facilitate our getting together. Once they arrive, we can begin the empowerment process.

Adult ADHD Group

David Wiggins, Ph.D., has begun offering a four-session psychoeducational group for adults who believe they may be ADHD. During these four sessions, the leaders present didactic material that generates discussion.

It was not originally designed to be a high-powered clinical intervention, but the people who attend love it. Most of them report: "We have never talked like this before!" They are thrilled, and many return for individual therapy. As a result of the success with this group, Dr. Wiggins is now making plans for an Adult ADHD Center. This Center will offer assessment, psychoeducational groups, adult/marital/family therapy, and consultation between client and, at the client's request, employer. (Dr. Wiggins has extensive training in rehabilitation.) Of course, once therapists have made a connection with an employer in regard to one individual, other reasons for consultation with that employer may arise. Marketing involves keeping your eyes open for opportunities.

ACOA Group

Louis A. Perrott, Ph.D., has been offering groups for adult children of alcoholics (ACOAs) for years. He is addressing his services to a topic of urgent concern to many people. Because he likes to do psychodrama, his groups are done within that mode. He offers groups that last 8–12 sessions. Members are helped to relate current behavior patterns with family of origin issues and then helped to work those issues through. Many members return for additional group series or for individual and marital work.

ACOA Parent Group

In response to the success of the ACOA group, Drs. Perrott and Lampron have just devised a group approach to helping ACOA parents with their own children. "Don't let it happen to your children" is the theme. The goal is to help people raised in alcoholic homes develop more functional child-rearing practices than were used with them. The ACOA Parent Group is offered on the basis that, unless people have developed alternatives, they are extremely likely to repeat patterns their own parents used. Parenting is an issue of urgent concern to many people, as is protecting their children from the particular horrors they endured as children themselves.

Breaking Away from Food Dependence

Mary Ann Koch, Ph.D., helps people with excess weight, almost all of whom have been through most of the countless weight-loss programs available today. This therapist, in partnership with a dietician, offers a time-limited (10 sessions) group approach that deals with the behavioral and psychological issues involved. The income for the group work is at market rates, and many of her satisfied clients return for other kinds of services.

OTHER UNMANAGED POSSIBILITIES

What follow are some non-DSM-oriented services that therapists can offer. Some of these services are currently being conducted, while others are still ideas. These services can be useful in and of themselves but also serve to introduce you to the community. As people experience you as helpful in one area of their lives, they are likely to call on you when other issues arise.

This list is not intended to be comprehensive. If you can use some of these ideas in your own practice, great! The main idea, however, is to stimulate your creativity. It is to remind you that, if you focus on issues of living rather than DSM diagnoses, your opportunities will be limited only by your imagination and your *willingness to follow through* (i.e., implementation).

Marriage Training

The divorce rate is soaring, but our society has yet to offer systematic ways of teaching the skills required to function well in a marriage. Churches might be particularly interested in sponsoring programs for engaged couples in their congregations. This could be a four-session program offered in the evenings to groups. Six couples or more at $25 per couple per meeting may make it financially acceptable for you. If these couples run into snags down the road, who are they going to call? When the clergy of that church run into marital problems in the congregation, who will they know who is knowledgeable about marriage? In fact, you and the clergy may create a strategic partnership between you. That builds tremendous referral power. Again, *marketing involves keeping your eyes open for opportunities*.

I reviewed this idea with my brother-in-law, a former clergyman. He liked the idea but offered a warning about an important factor I had overlooked. To maintain his position with his congregation, the clergyman cannot afford to be left out of such a program. Therefore, if you do this program, do not consign your host to a seat in the back of the room. Instead, offer your host an active role. Otherwise, your program might get rejected for reasons that you would never hear about. You may also need to negotiate a fee arrangement because the clergy will not be expected to charge for services. You could offer to donate a percentage of your fees to the church to help support ongoing educational programs.

This example illustrates a significant issue in developing niche services. The process requires a certain amount of armchair thinking, but don't stop there. Get out and talk with people about your ideas. Do some reality testing to keep you from including a fatal flaw in an otherwise sound plan.

Child and Family Stress

"Helping Children with Stress" is my old reliable PTA talk. Despite my having given this talk 50 times or more in my community over the past 15 years, it still gets requested and always goes over well. Parents usually stop me afterward to ask questions. I give handouts with my name and "10 tips" outlined. Copies of the edition of my newsletter that dealt with this topic have frequently been requested. The talk, handout, and newsletter all generate requests for services.

Therapists could develop a three-session child stress assessment *or* family stress assessment. This type of arrangement enables children, parents, and families to examine the stresses in their lives without having to wait until someone develops a DSM-IV diagnosable problem. (Stress is not considered shameful; if anything, it is seen as a badge of honor.) The three-session package would permit the participants to experience you, to see what these kinds of discussions are like, and to get some feedback from an expert about where they stand.

Adults and Stress

For adults, offer special services to the "stress-prone person." "Stress" is a word people understand, at least on an intuitive level. An introductory workshop followed up by group or individual consultations might be highly successful. It is an alternative to the stress management workshops offered by many employers. Invite people to "learn how stress affects your physical health now, before you develop serious problems." Encourage them to develop a relationship with a "stress coach" who can help to guide them away from life-shortening behaviors.

Children and Divorce

Divorced parents are almost always concerned about the effects of divorce on their children. A three-session assessment model can be developed to examine the child's view of and response to the process. Emphasize the fact that these services are for normal people going through a normal process. Parents are invited to call *before* symptoms become disruptive. In other words, you have not only created a nice entry-level service but also are practicing secondary prevention.

Facilitating the Emotional Divorce

What if it became as normal for divorcing people to consult therapists as to consult attorneys? People would get more for their money and have fewer problems. Develop a three- to four-session program for newly separated and divorced people. It could be done in a group format in which the normal aspects of the process are considered. Or it could be done in an individual assessment process. Some courts might be interested in promoting such interventions because they would cut down the hassle factor for them, not to mention helping divorcing individuals. Those who go through your program and want more service are likely to call you.

In addition, I read about an attorney who teamed up with a clinician. Tired of listening to his divorcing clients' emotional problems—about which he could do nothing—he arranged for a therapist to be available for those needs. The attorney is now free to handle the legal issues while the therapist handles the emotional ones. I recently consulted with a therapist/lawyer team who have used their partnership in this way with considerable success.

PMS Skills

There is a woman psychologist in Boulder, Colorado, whom I happened to see on the *Today Show*. She offers help on the subject of premenstrual syndrome (PMS). She works with individuals and groups offering a short-term assessment and treatment model. While she does not claim to make PMS go away, a properly prepared therapist can offer both the woman and her family some approaches to handling the difficulties more comfortably. My guess is that, if you are helpful, she or her family will seek out your services in the future on this or unrelated matters.

Sex Offenders

Psychotherapy Finances, in a recent edition, outlined programs for treating nonimprisoned sex offenders. Obviously, this type of program is not going to appeal to everyone. However, there is apparently a ready market, and the clients *must pay* or they go to jail. This example is not one that fits in with the "introductory" model. However, it does fit with the approach of speaking to issues of urgent concern. The urgent concern is: "How do I keep myself out of jail?"

Obviously, this work will require some focused preparation and training, but such a requirement is nothing new for us. We are accustomed to obtaining whatever additional training we need to provide new services in a professional manner.

Family Violence

This is a tough one. The need, however, is undeniable. Therapists who develop effective interventions in anger management/violent behavior will not need to worry about managed care. Think about some of the men who abuse their wives. They are often proud, rigid, and easily shamed. Their response to shame is violence. Today, in order to get services for their problem, more shame—the shame of being given a psychiatric diagnosis—is required. These rigid men often get out of treatment as soon as possible, with disappointing results. Might not some of them respond better to an approach that normalized their feelings and issues, though certainly not their behavior? Perhaps you could call the program "learning to love tenderly." After such a reorientation in thinking, a therapeutic alliance can be formed that can engender genuine behavior change.

The Quest for Meaning

Behind all the frenetic activity of modern life, people search to put meaning in their lives. To illustrate, pay never ranks number 1 in surveys regarding what people value in their jobs. Having meaningful work usually does. Think about it yourself. Couldn't you find a way to make more money than you can as a therapist, if money were your first priority? It is the meaning of the work to you that most likely is the key. People search for meaning in their work and in other aspects of their lives as well. We are particularly skilled at helping people find meaning in their lives. Those of us who find ways to communicate that as a service are likely to develop a strong clientele.

The Family Meal

Many families have lost the time-honored tradition of the dinner hour, normally a vital time for family bonding. Many family conflicts arise when attempts are made to recapture that time. A workshop or program focused on reestablishing that tradition is likely to have takers and is just as likely to lead to longer-term work.

Retreats for Lawyers

Attorneys experience a great deal of stress in their lives, not least of all owing to their low standing in the eyes of most Americans. A recent survey reported in our local paper indicated that a greater proportion of attorneys are depressed than is true among any of the other 102 professions studied; 1 lawyer in 10 thinks of suicide at least once per month.

A therapy group in the Hudson Valley in New York holds retreats for lawyers, designed for psychological renewal. There is even a group called The International Alliance of Holistic Lawyers. Attorneys need us. Those of us who are interested in forensic work will likely find this to be a wonderful practice-building tool. Designing similar retreats for other professional groups offers additional opportunities.

Prevention of Childhood Depression

Seligman (1990) has developed the concept of a "vaccine" against depression that can be used with children. He found that he could have a "very large effect" on 10- to 11-year-olds. My colleague Richard Milan, Ph.D., developed the following plan. Children could be screened for high risk of developing pessimistic/depressive patterns. Then candidates could be seen in groups of eight for two or more sessions, examining attribution style at an age-appropriate level. Didactic information delivered via role play and humor could be used. Marketing could be done through schools, churches, Boy Scouts, Girl Scouts, athletic organizations, and so on. However, you would not associate the term "depression" with this approach—you could call it "working with the pessimistic child." That would save you, the parents, and the children from the burden and barrier of psychiatric baggage.

Life Span Developmental Consultation

As mentioned earlier, Arthur Kovacs, Ph.D., a prominent psychologist in Los Angeles, has developed his practice by framing his services around helping people deal with the natural difficulties that occur during such transitions in life as marriage, divorce, graduation, retirement, the birth of children, and children leaving home. How many life transitions have you already helped people through? Was a DSM diagnosis really the best way to conceptualize the normal pain of transitions? If you use DSM criteria as the primary indicator for whether or not someone should be in therapy, you are in actuality making a decision that the client should be the one to make. With the exception of those who use therapy only to satisfy chronic dependency needs, people should be able to elect to see a therapist whenever they want to do so.

Grief Work with Parents Who Lose Children

This is an emotionally tough but deeply rewarding area. It is not an area for which I would have volunteered. However, when children within the families of my clients have died, those families asked for my help. I found it to be emotionally intense and deeply rewarding. Gerald Koocher (1994) has developed a program to help those parents. It is an issue of urgent concern but not short term work.

Consultation with Clergy

More people consult clergy about personal problems than any other kind of professional. Consider offering an hour or two of consultation per month to a group of clergy, helping them to build their skills in responding to these requests. The benefits include upgrading the skills of a highly stressed group, likely access to a large number of referrals as they recognize those parishioners whose problems are beyond their ability to help, and perhaps therapy services to many clergymen and clergywomen themselves.

Vehicle Therapy

No, this does not mean giving up your practice to become a mechanic. A group of therapists in New York City has bought a fleet of vans and hired drivers. The therapists see clients, mostly highly stressed executive types, on their way to or from work.

Smoking Cessation

It's not new, but it works. There are still a lot of smokers out there. Increasing pressure to stop smoking is having the effect of making this an issue of urgent concern. There are a variety of one- to four-session programs on the market. This is a good entry-level service.

Divorce Mediation

A therapist in the Washington, D.C., area told me that "divorce mediation won't work as a practice-building technique up here. Everybody's doing it." Okay. So, do it better. Or put a different twist on it. Network better. Market better.

You will run into a gazillion naysayers. That happens to people who challenge conventional wisdom. In this case, conventional wisdom is that if you are not on 15 managed care panels you might as well start mowing lawns. Your willingness to have hope and courage challenges the decisions that naysayers make in response to their own anxiety and despair.

Psychological Hardiness

In Chapter 4 we reviewed the three C's of psychological hardiness: Teach them. They have unlimited applications. People who are seriously ill, executives going through major upheavals in their companies, and families going through the stresses of major changes in their lives could all benefit. Psychological hardiness is a life skill that is universally useful.

Again, this list of suggestions is mainly intended to get you thinking about the possibilities once we let go of the medical model and begin thinking about human problems. Review the results of your three free market studies to see what gets sparked within your own imagination.

SUMMARY

Use of the Problem-Solving/Skill-Building model enables us to approach service development in ways that are creative and responsive to the needs and interests of all people in our society. By knowing their issues and speaking their language, we can increase the likelihood that we will be seen as valuable. By offering a variety of attractive, unthreatening ways for people to begin talking with us, we can enter into relationships much more easily. Then, once they learn something about us and our methods, people will be in a much better position to evaluate whether further sessions will be of value to them. These strategies go a long way toward overcoming the barriers that have too long existed between us and potential clients.

Chapter 7

Planning the Business of Your Practice

This chapter will help you make a business plan for your practice. The chapter largely consists of a series of questions with discussion to guide you. At the end of the chapter is a form you can use to record your answers to the questions. Take a moment to review the form (see Box 7.6 on pages 140–142) so you have a sense of what is coming. Then, taking all the time you need, work through this chapter. When you have read through the chapter and answered the questions, you will have a well-constructed plan that will offer guidance through the often difficult and confusing days ahead.

WHAT BUSINESS ARE YOU IN?

Answering this question is the first step in creating a business plan. It is not enough to say that you are in the therapy business. The word "therapy" is too broad and nonspecific for our purposes. Defining your particular business means determining the actual services you plan to provide. Doing so sharpens your thinking and lays the foundation for the rest of your plan.

Part I of this book provides a conceptual framework with which to start considering what business you are in. The key points now are (1) to remember the value of your work and (2) to let go of the medical model in favor of integrating the concepts of the Problem-Solving/Skill-Building model with your own favorite theoretical school(s).

Chapters 5 and 6 provided some key elements in shaping your list of

113

services. Chapter 5 spoke about the three key strategies: (1) people respond to their own urgent concerns, (2) people buy on the basis of benefits, not features, and (3) people need an easy way to start. Chapter 6 outlined ways to determine the urgent concerns people in your community may have. It also provided examples of services that fit our criteria.

As you define your business, also consider this. My plan is to be able to work in my community for the next couple of decades. I assume you have a similar time table. Therefore, the opportunities we will find must be based on providing quality services and long term satisfaction for both our clients and ourselves.

Now, in preparation for defining the nature of your business, make four lists. Your first list will be the results of your market studies (see Box 7.1). What are the issues that appear to be of urgent concern to people within the community you plan to serve? Many of these issues may be of universal concern, such as child rearing and marital issues. However, your community may also emphasize particular issues. For example, areas with large immigrant communities may have concerns related to acculturation, whereas rural communities may have issues related to the economic and social impact of the passing of family farms. If you live in a community dominated by a military base, which means that the average period of residence in your community may be 18 months, offering long-term psychoanalytic therapy is unlikely to get many takers, no matter how good you are.

Next, make a list of the kinds of services you are *interested in* providing (see Box 7.2). For the moment, do not worry about whether you are

---

BOX 7.1. Results of Market Studies: Issues of Urgent Concern

1. _____
2. _____
3. _____
4. _____
5. _____
6. _____
7. _____
8. _____
9. _____
10. _____

BOX 7.2. Services That Command My Interest

1. _____
2. _____
3. _____
4. _____
5. _____
6. _____
7. _____
8. _____
9. _____
10. _____

---

trained to give these services, because you can always get more training. Right now, we are just looking at your interests, what excites you. "Doing psychodrama" is not an appropriate entry for this list. Psychodrama is a method, not a service. If you like doing psychodrama, great. How do you want to use that method? Decide on the life issues for which you believe psychodrama (or psychoanalysis, or cognitive–behavior modification, or whatever) to be appropriate and list them.

You may find yourself writing down life issues expressed in the technical terms of your favorite school(s) of therapy. That is an acceptable beginning. However, once you have done *that* list, translate it into everyday language. This act of translation is important for two reasons. First, translating the issues into simpler language ensures that you are thinking clearly. It is a good test of our own understanding of a concept to be able to translate it from technical language into everyday language. Second, one day you will want to communicate with potential candidates for your services. Almost none of those people went to graduate school to learn therapy jargon. Translating your list now will help to ensure that you are not creating unnecessary barriers to people reaching you.

The third list that can help you define your business is a list of the services you are currently trained to provide (see Box 7.3). This list will include those services you currently provide and perhaps additional services that, for various reasons, you may not currently offer. For example, although I am thoroughly trained in psychometric testing relevant to identifying emotional conflicts, I do much less testing these days than I used to do. This is just an evolutionary aspect of my particular practice. Yet,

---

BOX 7.3. Services I Am Trained to Do

1. _____
2. _____
3. _____
4. _____
5. _____
6. _____
7. _____
8. _____
9. _____
10. _____

---

because it is something I am trained to do, it would be on my list as "psychometric testing relevant to identifying emotional conflicts."

As with the previous list, this list will not be a list of methods. Instead, the items will speak to life issues or specific applications. "Providing behavioral therapy for premature ejaculation" would be an entry, whereas "behavioral therapy" by itself would not be.

Finally, there is one more list to write. This is a list of those services that fall within our general field but that you choose *not* to provide (see Box 7.4). Sometimes we get offered work we do not want. That may sound unlikely if you are scrambling to make your next mortgage payment. Yet, it is true. Part of defining what businesses you are in is determining what business you are not in. This decision may be based on training, expertise, and/or personal preferences. Work we do not want consumes time and energy, preventing those *key resources* from being used more productively.

In my case, there are a variety of things I choose not to do. Obviously, I choose not to be on managed care provider panels. There have been numerous opportunities to join such panels that I have declined. Of course, that does not happen much any more. Whatever options I might have once had in that area are long gone. Likewise, I do not work with people willing to be held prisoner by insurance company rules. When those rules interfere with my provision of effective services, I ask clients to make a choice.

He was 17, with an IQ higher than mine. It would be generous to call his academic record spotty. When he was about to enter his senior year, his parents brought him to therapy to become prepared to suc-

---

BOX 7.4. Services I Choose Not to Offer

1. _____
2. _____
3. _____
4. _____
5. _____
6. _____
7. _____
8. _____
9. _____
10. _____

---

ceed in college. He had carried a diagnosis of ADHD since he began school. It had become a part of how he identified himself. It also was a part of how his parents identified him. The family's way of understanding ADHD made it impossible to reach the appropriate therapy goals for which they sought my services. Part of the therapeutic task was to reorient everyone's vision of this soon-to-be-man from one of handicap to one of competence. Otherwise, he would never give himself permission to do what he must to succeed in college. Before we could do that, we had to help the family see how the parents' years of helping were now creating barriers to growth. This took some time and involved individual and family sessions.

After about two months of weekly appointments, in which some progress was made, his parents said they wanted our appointments to be every other week. Their insurance would pay for only 25 visits per year, and they wanted to stretch out our work in order to prevent running out of benefits. In this case, I did not believe the frequency they requested was sufficient to meet our goals.

I had us review our goals. Reasonable consensus was reached. I then explained that I could not help them meet their goals within the artificial constraints created by limits on insurance benefits, adding: "If you want someone willing to work within those rules, I would be happy to help you find another therapist." The parents initially looked at me with some shock. However, they knew that their son had become invested in therapy and that our direction made sense. The parents elected to continue as we had been, and everyone's commitment to our work deepened.

Working with families with unresolved sexual abuse allegations is work I find unpleasant. I refer such offers to practitioners who have the emotional energy for them. While I like helping people recover from divorce, I do not enjoy custody evaluations. During initial interviews, I make it clear that I can be the family's therapist or I can be involved in court actions, but not both. Those who want me primarily as a weapon in court, under the guise of therapist, usually find someone else. Some other people switch goals, deciding what they really want is a therapist.

Now review these four lists. What items are common to lists 1, 2, and 3 but do not show up on list 4? Those common items are the core of your new practice. Make a separate list of them. You can always expand your services in the future by getting more training or developing new interests or by learning of new needs in your community. However, for now, these services define your business.

Take a final check of your core list. Do these services pass the tests for a private pay practice? Are they based on issues that are of real concern to potential consumers? Are they expressed in language that people in your target audience would readily understand? Are some of them entry-level or introductory services?

WRITE A MISSION STATEMENT

A mission statement is a *brief* statement that describes what your practice is about. It is the absolute core of your purpose. Writing a good mission statement will force you to think clearly about what you are doing and why, and about the values you have that underlie your work. It will force you to think clearly because it can only be about three sentences long, yet it has to communicate to anyone who cares to read it what you are about.

How do you know what your mission is? Having constructed these four lists—not an easy task—helps to prepare you to write a mission statement for your practice. Review your core list of services. Ask yourself why each item is there. Why is it important to you to offer those particular services? Also pay close attention to list 4, those services you choose not to provide. They may also speak to your values and mission. As you construct your mission statement, you can test its soundness by examining how it fits with your list of core services.

Your mission statement may be several hours—or even several months—in the making. It is not easy to think so clearly. The process that creates a good mission statement is worth whatever time and energy are required, because it is that thinking that will guide you during inevitable periods of doubt and confusion.

I once served on a committee for one of our professional organizations. The chair of the committee submitted a mission statement for our review. It was two pages long! Calling it a mission statement did not make it one. It contained background, justification, and strategies. You may in fact find it useful to create a document that includes all that material—it's a way of organizing thought that works for some people. However, the mission statement is what is distilled from that exercise, not the exercise itself.

Thus, your initial try may be considerably longer than one to three sentences. As my editor taught me, writers usually need a lot more words to get their message on paper initially than they will keep in the long run.

The mission statement for the part of my practice devoted to traditional services is: "To provide services to children, adolescents, families, and adults of sufficient depth, length, and thoughtfulness that clients solve developmental problems and build needed skills." Embedded within this one sentence is a great deal of information. It identifies my potential clients. It expresses my passionate belief that outside, artificial constraints will not guide my work, but rather guidance will come from the client and myself. Finally, it places my work squarely within the Problem-Solving/Skill-Building model.

IDENTIFYING AND ASSESSING YOUR COMPETITION

Having identified the services you offer, you need to begin to recognize who else can or does provide services that address the same urgent concerns of your potential clients. These are your competitors. They seek the same funds that are drawing your attention. While only you can identify the specific competitors in your area, they will probably tend to fall into the following groups.

Other private pay clinicians. Some competitors will be other private pay oriented therapists. As you will see, you *want* some of this competition.

Managed care. Another set of competitors are managed care based therapists. Thus far, I have wanted to minimize managed care as a competitor because therapists have paid too much attention to the moves managed care makes, and because we really offer quite different packages. However, because they and we seem to be relatively undifferentiated in the public's mind, they do represent some competition. Much of this is a language problem, since each camp is fond of using the word "therapy." Yet, we mean quite different things by it. The public must be forgiven for not understanding the distinctions right now. We have some educating to do.

Other competition. The public also looks to other sources of help. Our competitors include public agencies, the clergy, physicians, and attorneys. Attorneys?! Yes. For example, should a couple hire you to help them with their marital problems or hire attorneys to get a divorce? Should a family hire attorneys to fight a custody battle, or should they hire people like us to help promote emotional healing?

WHAT ADVANTAGES DO YOU HAVE OVER YOUR OTHER COMPETITORS?

When compared to many of our competitors, our depth of training and experience provide a clear advantage. It is important for you to recognize these differences as you plan your business. However, as you will see in Chapter 8, we will not use marketing techniques that disparage others. Doing so is not only unprofessional but also bad for business. You will *not* gain business by bad-mouthing others. However, by understanding your advantages, you can find ways to highlight your strengths. In addition, as you examine the strengths and weaknesses of yourself and your competition, you can find ways to *work with your competitors* for your mutual advantage. As Jay Conrad Levinson, author of *Guerrilla Marketing,* says: "I don't have competitors. Just allies" (Yudkin, 1994, p. 27).

Primary Care Physicians

Most physicians use the medical model. We can choose not to. When we step outside the medical model, our ability to be creative in our ways of understanding human problems provides flexibility in responding to those problems. Primary care physicians do not have their practices organized so that they have time to sit with someone an hour a week for many weeks or months. Moreover, the amount of time that frontline physicians will be able to devote to listening to their patients will probably decline further with the near-term advance of managed care.

How can we work together? Primary care physicians will not have your breadth of training in therapy. Physicians want to give their patients what they need but often do not have the resources to provide it. Physicians who work in a capitated system may be reluctant to refer their patients directly to a therapist. However, if you have a private pay practice, referring to you does not affect a physician's compensation. If you develop a brochure outlining the advantages of coming to see you, the physician may pass your brochure on to his or her patients — and possibly make referrals, as well. By referring the patient to you, the physician becomes an *indirect* source of what the patient needs. The patient gets what he or she needs and is satisfied with the physician's response to the problem.

Clergy

Clergy are consulted about human problems more often than any other professionals (and they are not battling managed care!). However, many in the clergy have told me that they get too little training in responding to such problems. For example, they report little education or guidance in setting *appropriate* boundaries between themselves and their parishioners. The culture's expectations of the clergy make it difficult for them to set limits on their availability.

How can we work together? To their parishioners the clergy may seem like endless sources of comfort, but being so available is bound to be extremely stressful. If you form a good relationship with a local clergyman or clergywoman, you may become colleagues rather than competitors. You may find ways to work together with troubled members of the congregation, which in and of itself will provide great support to the clergy. Your use of the Problem-Solving/Skill-Building model makes it much easier for the clergy to make referrals to you, because the emotional barriers created by the mental illness model are totally absent.

Public Agencies

Public agencies get the toughest cases despite having the fewest resources. Often their staff are entry-level therapists because experienced therapists have either moved into private practice or been elevated to administration. People who can afford to see a private therapist usually will. You have clear advantages of flexibility, privacy, and expertise.

How can we work together? If, as we discussed in Chapter 3, your therapy community is successful in shaping a public clinic to the Problem-Solving/Skill-Building model with reduced-fee subsidized private pay, you will have a good place to refer clients who want to pay out of pocket but cannot afford your fee. Donating a portion of your workweek to the clinic is also one way to satisfy any wish to provide pro bono services.

Attorneys

When one compares our services to those offered by lawyers, we have many advantages. For example, people often try to settle "who was right" in a marriage via an expensive divorce proceeding in the courts. We know that often such a process may only intensify the emotional entanglements and won't necessarily settle matters long term. To move past a divorce, people must sever their emotional connections in a struggle to achieve not vindication, but detachment. By definition, it is impossible to be detached within the adversarial system. We know how to facilitate marital negotiation and compromise, and our fees are usually far less than attorneys' fees. The value of a better outcome for less money is hard to beat.

How can we work together? Attorneys, like physicians and the clergy, want to give their clients what they really need. Doing so is only good business. However, they often do not have the time or the expertise to do so. Their time is better spent litigating in court, not settling marital disputes. As we discussed earlier (see page 108), an attorney/therapist combination is a natural because clients get better service while attornies are saved from emotional hassles and from providing difficult-to-bill-for services.

Managed Care

In head-to-head competition with managed care, we have many advantages. We can offer genuine privacy. Client and therapist control treatment. Services are individualized, not designed by a manual. Clients need not suffer the burdens of a psychiatric diagnosis. Our flexibility in designing interventions is much greater. People do not have to be "crazy" to see us.

How we can work together? Our model is of course not compatible with the managed care model, so there is really no way to work with managed care per se. However, there is a way to work with therapists who are on managed care panels, who work within capitated systems, or who work for a vertically integrated monopoly. Let's suppose someone goes to see a therapist and uses managed care just because that is what they have and they do not know about the disadvantages. Then suppose something goes wrong. Maybe they are not considered "crazy enough," and treatment is not authorized. Or maybe their sessions run out too soon, or they want something deeper than brief therapy and medication. Or perhaps they ask about the privacy issue and do not like what they hear.

This therapist is now in a bind. Like other professionals, the therapist wants to give the client what the client wants or needs but he or she does not have the resources at hand to do so. This therapist could refer the client to you. You could set up referral relationships to be activitated in situations such as these. Since you have a private pay practice, the managed care therapist could refer to you without fear of sanctions. The client would get what is needed, and you would have a referral.

Other Therapists

Many of the advantages we may have when compared to other private pay therapists who offer similar services to our own have to do with practical issues. For example, the American Psychological Association, at the

State Leadership Training Conference in 1993, reported on a study they had done about how people chose a therapist. The most powerful factor identified was whether the therapist provided convenient parking! So there you are, having spent years in training and supervision, going to workshops, painstakingly developing a set of ethical, powerful interventions. And what determines whether all that preparation and training will pay off is . . . asphalt!

This finding reminds us that we are in a *customer service business.* We need to consider the comfort and convenience issues of our clients — certainly our competition will. These issues include parking, secretarial/ receptionist services, location, and your accessibility. These practical considerations can help you to differentiate yourself from your competitors.

At the Manassas Group, we value our secretarial and receptionist staff highly. They are our face to the public. How they treat our clients has a major impact on our relationships with our clients. How they greet *potential* clients, calling for the first time, has a powerful impact on whether a first appointment actually happens. Among the chief secrets of our success are that we pay higher staff salaries, do more careful hiring, and provide more training in relating to the public than do our competitors. When we hire someone, we ask ourselves:

- Can this person remain composed and courteous even when a client does not?
- Can this person maintain a friendly attitude while (usually simultaneously) three lines are ringing, two clients at the front desk are waiting to schedule, and one of the therapists is asking for attention?
- Can this person keep matters confidential (e.g., resisting the pressure to reveal whether someone's spouse or former spouse has an appointment with us)?
- Can this person ask for payment with courtesy and firmness?

Our clients frequently comment on the friendliness and helpfulness of our front office staff, indicating that we enjoy a huge advantage over our competition in this regard.

> I returned a call from a therapist who had inquired about some managed care free practice issues. I reached his answering machine, and listend to a tape made by, I assume, his secretary. She said: "If you want to leave a message for Dr. W., please press '1' on your touch-tone phone. If you do not have a touch-tone phone, it is time to get one!" A derisive attitude like this toward those who pay your bills is poison to your practice.

How can we work together? While other private pay therapists are your most direct competition, they are also your greatest allies. A little-known fact of business is that competition breeds business. The more you and other therapists in your area spread the gospel that (1) everybody has problems, (2) tackling them head-on feels good, and (3) private pay is worth the money and then some, the larger you have made the private pay market for everybody. Toward this end, you may want to band together with other private pay therapists to establish a marketing guild to promote your public education campaign. (Ivan Miller, Ph.D., in Boulder, Colorado, has done just that — see the Appendix for his address and phone number.)

Also, remember the buddy system. Most of us who are swimming upstream against conventional wisdom will need the companionship and support of other therapists. What one person cannot seem to get off the ground, two sometimes can. Form strategic partnerships with other therapists around the development of particular services. You do not *have* to be in business together to do this, but you could be. Other private pay therapists can refer people to you and your special services. You can return the favor. What we are looking for is collegial and congenial competition that leads therapists to make appropriate referrals and provide consultation to one another.

WHAT ABOUT YOUR COMPETITORS' ADVANTAGES?

You do not hold all the cards. No one does. Your competitors have advantages over you. If you know those advantages, you can plan around them.

Physicians and the clergy have both prestige and a sense of normalcy as advantages. We hope eventually to share that sense of normalcy with them, but we have not gotten there yet. These are better established professions than ours. People are used to going to them for help. Because they have been helpful in some matters, medical or spiritual, people hope they can get other kinds of help from them too. Further, people do not have to confront the shame and stigma of mental illness by going to these professionals. While they will not have to deal with those issues with us either, *people do not yet know that.*

Physicians and managed care practitioners have the advantage of insurance reimbursement. While we know that people pay a steep price for that advantage, it is an advantage nonetheless. We have ways of overcoming that advantage, as we have discussed.

Physicians have a perceived advantage of access to psychotropic medication. While the literature (as reviewed in Chapter 2), does not support medication as a long-term solution for most people, many people currently see it as quicker, cheaper, and easier. The answer is for us to educate the public about the advantages and effectiveness of our approaches.

To be clear, I do not mean to suggest that psychotropic medications are never appropriate. There are times to add medications to the treatment mix. Sometimes, intervening at the chemical level of the system increases our effectiveness. However, that approach has been oversold to our culture and our profession. Using the Problem-Solving/Skill-Building model can help us to reestablish an appropriate balance.

SETTING PRICES

Pricing products and services is an issue that all businesses must handle. A basic tenet of business practice is that prices must cover the real costs of doing business. Several factors need to be considered, including your costs in running a practice, your own income goals, your competitors' pricing, and the value of your services.

Costs

Your costs include a host of things: office rent or mortgage payments, office staff wages, payroll taxes, paper, pencils, electricity, telephone, copying, malpractice and office liability insurance, postage, etc. Consider these costs seriously. If you work with adolescents, you know that, for various reasons, many are eager to move out of their home and live on their own. You also know from talking to them that they have little concept of the amount of money they will need to cover their costs. Yet, we often have set up shop without doing our homework on costs.

You need to be able to predict your expenses. Otherwise, you may think that you are making plenty of money, only to find that not much of it gets into your pocket. Box 7.5 lists most of the expenses you are likely to encounter. The bulk of this list is adapted by permission from a wonderful book by Mark Lewin (1978), who wrote a primer on starting a private practice that was of immense help to me and is still relevant today.

Your Income

You also must decide how much money you want or need to generate as income. How much must you net from your practice to make it worth your while? This question is likely to resurrect the internal conflicts that we often have about money (discussed in Chapter 3). If you find yourself struggling with setting your financial goals, reread that section (pages 31–46).

BOX 7.5. Estimated Expenses of an Office Practice

Therapist's FICA	$_____
Office staff's net wages (take-home pay)	_____
Office staff's FICA	_____
Payroll withholding taxes (federal and state)	_____
Unemployment insurance	_____
Office rent/mortgage	_____
Office cleaning and maintenance	_____
Office supplies	_____
Professional supplies	_____
Professional memberships, books, and journals	_____
Continuing education and professional meetings	_____
Postage	_____
Telephone	_____
Utilities	_____
Marketing	_____
Travel	_____
Professional liability insurance	_____
Medical insurance	_____
Income protection insurance	_____
Comprehensive fire, theft, office liability insurance	_____
Life insurance	_____
Professional services (legal and accounting)	_____
Pension or 401-K Plan payments	_____
Depreciation on office furniture and equipment	_____
Miscellaneous (gifts, business lunches, charity)	_____
Total	$_____

Remember that the amount of income you desire is your own business. Steel yourself against the agendas that some people may have about what income is appropriate for you. They do not have to live with the consequences of your decisions. Therefore, they do not get to make them. If you do not make the kind of income you deserve, you communicate your belief that your services lack value. If you earn less than you *believe* you deserve, you will become resentful, and it will show.

A woman in one of our seminars talked of treating seriously emotionally disturbed children. She had done so for years with satisfaction. Lately she found that she was tired and dispirited. She had little energy for the children who now came to see her. She knew her work was affected and was giving serious thought to leaving the profession.

What had changed? Managed care was now seeing to it that her income had fallen well below the level she believed she was worth. Until the seminar, she had not given herself permission to see the link between her energy level and her income. When she did, she could begin to make plans to earn the kind of money she needed in order to have energy again. Rather than leave the profession, she saw that she could still provide services to children through a private pay practice.

Competitors' Pricing

If you charge double what others charge for the same service, you may have difficulty convincing people that your value is double. On the other hand, if you charge a lot less than your competition, you may be sending a message that either your self-esteem is low or that the value of your services is less than that of your competitors. In addition, you could be leaving a lot of money on the table that could have been in your pocket. I have given myself a raise every few years. The raise covers inflation in my business costs and in the cost of living. It also reflects the fact that, as I gain more experience, my services have greater value to my clients. People who are employed usually expect a raise every year or two for much the same reasons.

The UCRs that various insurance carriers set are less relevant than you may think. Do not use them to set your fees. Letting insurance companies establish our value is like asking a cereal company to set our fees. UCRs reflect only the amount that the insurance company is willing to part with to reimburse you for your services. Insurance companies do not receive the benefit of your services personally, nor do they know you. They do not have the necessary knowledge base to place a value on your particular services.

Managed care rates should *by no means* be used as a fee setting guide. Not only do the reasons above apply to managed care as well, but also your services are in a different category than the services managed care provides. If you match the managed care rates, you are marketing on the basis of comparative cost, not value. At the same time you are sending the misleading message to consumers that your services have value only equivalent to that of managed care services.

Estimating Income Realistically

Part of establishing your pricing relies on the number of billable hours available to you each year. Figure out how many billable hours you project in a year and then multiply that number by your hourly fee. The result will be an estimate of your annual gross income.

Before I began to diversify, when my clinical practice was all I did, I used the following formula. I figured I could count on being available 44 weeks out of 52. That left 8 weeks unbilled, which may seem high. If I was going to make a mistake, I wanted to underestimate my gross income, not live in a fantasy world. Those 8 weeks of unbilled time covered a variety of events and circumstances. I knew that I would take vacations, have holidays, go to conferences, do pro bono or volunteer work, and maybe get sick sometimes. I learned that I needed some time for practice-building activities. In addition, I knew that clients would sometimes miss appointments, not pay, or it would snow too much for anyone to get to the office, including me. I accounted for all those contingencies with those 8 weeks.

Then I had to figure out what a week's worth of billings really was. In my early days of full-time private practice, I billed 40 hours per week. Within 3 years I was burning out. I cut back from eight to seven clients per day. Eventually, I blocked off Wednesday mornings. I would do paperwork, reading, or write reports. Then I would go into the office at noon, staying late to run an evening group. This gave me 32 therapy hours per week plus a group that averaged five to seven clients per meeting.

Translating this into a formula using today's dollars: ([32 hours × $95/hour] + [6 clients × $50/group session]) × 44 weeks told me that I could expect to gross about $146,960 in a year. That was a useful piece of information! With that I could plan an office budget, know what I could afford to spend on various office expenses, and what I could then look forward to taking home. My gross income would sometimes vary from this estimate, which is all right. It still gave me a measuring stick against which I could assess how I was doing financially.

Remember to consider *the value of your services*. Review Chapter 2. Use the information there to remind yourself about the clinical and economic value that your services have. Take your level of education, your licenses and certifications, any specialized training, and your level of experience into account. This approach provides a much more realistic foundation for estimating your worth than the guilt and conflicted feelings about money that we have long been subject to, in part reflecting a unique occupational hazard.

FINANCIAL POLICIES

The discussion of price setting sets the stage to establish the financial policies you will use with your clients. It is important to establish a fee struc-

ture and collections policies ahead of time because you will be pressured
to make compromises. If those pressures come at a time you are sweating
the mortgage payment, you may find yourself making decisions that you
later come to regret.

> My brother, Roger, has two daughters, Annette and Michelle, both
> now grown, married, and delightful. During their teen years, however,
> Roger, like any father, worried about what might happen on dates,
> and he knew his daughters might object to his tagging along. There-
> fore, he had to arm them as best he could beforehand. Among the
> things he told them was that the time to decide whether they would
> have sex was before the date, not when they were feeling pressured
> by the boy or their own desires. In other words, he suggested that
> they think things through ahead of time rather than responding to
> the pressure of the moment.

That's pretty good advice. We should use it, too.

Figure out now what you are going to charge. Know your rationale.
Figure out now when you expect payment. At time of service? Monthly?
When the client gets around to it? Decide what payment plans, if any,
you are comfortable using. As we noted earlier, helping professionals are
notoriously confused and ambivalent about money and its proper place
in life. We need to work through these feelings so that we can have consistent, businesslike financial policies. Remember, if we allow clients to
be financially irresponsible with us, we are treating them like children.
Such an approach is therapeutically unsound.

You may think that the most serious obstacle to providing therapy
services outside managed care is the loss of third-party reimbursement.
In truth, the biggest obstacles are the attitudes we ourselves have about
money and our services. The good and bad news is that our most difficult
challenge is within ourselves. Once our thoughts and emotions are clear,
the payment process can work much more smoothly. Unless people pay
us, we cannot stay in practice.

Today, most people *can* afford therapy, especially if financial arrangements can be made. When people are made aware of psychotherapy's clinical and economic value most of them become willing to rearrange their
priorities to make room for therapy in their budgets. We have long believed that private pay therapy is only for the rich. The $114 billion that
people spend out-of-pocket for unreimbursed health care services (Pelletier, 1993) belies that belief.

Still, if we abruptly begin demanding full payment out of pocket at
the time of service from every client, many might stop therapy while
others might not start. We can offer clients a variety of approaches to payment. Offering various payment plans widens our accessibility to people.

This is one way private pay can become accessible to the broad middle class.

What follows are some alternative payment plans. I have been using some of these plans and have found the great majority of clients to be favorably inclined to one alternative or another. Their relative responsiveness seems to be determined more by their interest in therapy than by their level of family income.

> She was a single mother with two teenagers and a low average income. All three people in the family needed the opportunity to examine their family stressors. She could have used her insurance but chose not to. She preferred to pay out of pocket to safeguard her children's privacy, rearranging her budget in response to the value she saw in the service.

Alternative Payment Plans

Each of the following alternatives was reviewed by my CPA and by my attorney, who also has a master's degree in health care administration. However, the prudent therapist will seek advice from his or her own attorney and CPA before using any of these plans.

Discounts

Offer a small administrative discount for not using insurance. The financial advantages to you are that your office resources are not expended in filing insurance claims, you do not have to send bills, and you do not have to wait for your money. The downside is that you lose whatever amount you discount. However, consider this a business expense rather than a loss. It is an expense of a new way of doing business that will draw in far more clients, at a higher rate, than doing business the managed care way.

The discount need not be large. In my experience, offering a $5 discount seems to be quite satisfactory. In fact, this is far and away the most popular plan among my private pay clients. That small discount seems to make a large emotional impact on clients' attitudes.

You may be concerned that insurance companies would argue that you are changing your UCR. Would they lower what they reimburse you for the claims you still file? Even worse, would they charge you with fraud? The answer is "No" to both questions if you approach the matter in a businesslike manner. Charge the client your *full fee* and then discount whatever you choose. Show it all on paper.

You will notice that managed care firms and insurance-sponsored preferred provider organizations (PPOs) are asking for discounts all the time. We have the right to offer discounts to whomever we choose, for whatever reasons we want. We do, however, need to show the full fee and have a coherent policy about offering discounts.

I do not favor large discounts, that is, matching what managed care would like to set as our fee. What we do has so much value that it sends the wrong message to offer steep discounts. However, that is a personal belief. Some of you may find this kind of discount appealing. There was a recent report in *Psychotherapy Finances* ("Practice Issues," 1995) of a husband and wife team of therapists who opened their joint practices two years ago. They too decided to avoid the managed care system. They began charging $40 per hour but only to get themselves established. They gradually raised their fees until they recently reached the $90 level. They combined this approach with active and effective marketing.

Sliding Scale Fees

Arthur Kovacs (personal communication, 1993) has developed a sophisticated approach to sliding scale fees. In 1992, his charges varied in $10 increments from $30 per session to $160 per session, based on income and whether the person was using insurance reimbursement. He integrates this plan with his "Life Span Developmental Perspective" approach to therapy, in which people consult him at critical points over their lifetimes. As years go by, people typically are making more money and pay higher fees for subsequent consultations.

The advantage of this approach is that it does make therapy more affordable to those at the lower end of the economic scale. That gets people in the door and appeals to the social conscience of many in our profession. One downside is that the more well-to-do are asked to subsidize other people's therapy. Some clients may object to this, preferring just to pay for their own. Their social conscience may operate differently (not worse) from ours. However, if the sliding scale information is given to all clients, not just the financially troubled, everyone can make his or her own decisions.

Another potential disadvantage of a sliding scale is getting overloaded with clients on the lower end of the scale, creating a serious economic problem for you. A few therapists have reported to me on this issue, saying that, for them, this did not turn out to be the case. The determining factor may have been their ways of marketing their practice. If you market in a way that appeals primarily to people at the low end of the income scale, you could have a problem.

Scholarships

A variation on the sliding scale idea would be to create a limited number of slots for those paying a lower fee. It would be like a college scholarship based on need. You could structure your approach by extending the analogy. People are accustomed to applying for college aid, so the concept is in place. Here, people could write an essay about how they would use the therapy experience to improve their lives. Hard work and continuing progress would be necessary to keep the scholarship. Otherwise, it would go to someone else who would make better use of it. The client could continue to see you but at your regular rate. If you choose to offer scholarships, be sure to work the cost of these slots into your financial plan.

Installment Plans

This is not a brand-new idea and yet it seems to be underused. Charge your regular fee but negotiate how much of that fee will be paid at the time of service (or monthly if that is how you bill). The balance would build over the course of treatment. At the end of treatment, the client makes monthly payments until the balance is satisfied.

I personally like this plan a lot better than offering deep discounts to people who find paying the entire fee each week unmanageable. By charging your normal fee but allowing clients to spread out the payments, you leave them in the adult position of paying their full amount. You also avoid the danger of hidden resentments on your part toward clients who require extra effort but provide smaller amounts of income.

The disadvantage of this plan is that you must wait to have use of the money. You are basically making a loan. One solution is to limit the amount of credit you will extend. My limit is $1,000, which gets clients through 20 sessions, since I require 50% payment at the time of visit. Then, if clients still need additional therapy, they arrange additional credit elsewhere. Repayment does not begin until therapy is completed. Payments are made in the same monthly amount people were making during their therapy. This has become the second favorite of three plans that I offer, but it is a distant second.

We spoke earlier of how such plans can make therapy accessible to the broad middle class. This particular plan offers one way for you to charge your full fee while also making your services available to most, though not all, people. Remember that 90% of episodes of care last less than 25 sessions. The Roanoke therapy rate is approximately $95 per session. If I see a client once every 2 weeks, on average, and collect 50% of the fee at the time of visit and then spread remaining payments out over the year following therapy, the client needs to be able to pay only about $100 per month. While there are some people in our society who would find that amount impossible, the vast majority will not.

The question of charging interest arises with this plan. Again, this *is* a loan. Charging interest would cover the interest you may be paying for money you are using while waiting for payments. You are either borrowing money or at least foregoing interest you could earn on investments.

My CPA points out that, with professional fees, people just do not like to pay interest. Thus, while there is nothing legally or morally wrong with charging interest, it can create relationship problems. He proposes (and himself uses) a compromise, charging interest but waiving interest charges as long as people are making agreed-upon principal payments in a timely manner. This keeps people motivated to make payments because, if they do not, you are free to invoke the interest charge.

If you follow that plan, be sure to consult a CPA or attorney regarding what interest rate to charge. You do not want to violate the usury laws in your state. Our CPA charges 2% per month, though the more normal rate is 1.5% per month. His rationale is that he is not trying to make money off interest. He is using that charge as a motivator to get people to honor their financial commitment.

A participant in one of my seminars wrote to give us a helpful modification. Dr. Harry Corsover said that he had been advised to frame this as a "late payment charge" rather than as an interest charge. It is a more straightforward approach, getting the message across more clearly. He has been charging interest for balances not paid within 60 days of billing.

Modified Orthodontist Plan

This plan is based on my experience with orthodontists for each of my three children. In this approach, the first four to six sessions are billed at your regular fee, preferably on a pay-as-you-go basis. This gives you an opportunity to assess the client's needs and formulate a treatment plan.

You can then negotiate to provide all needed services, within negotiated limits, over a specific number of months for a specified fee. For example, suppose a client needs weekly sessions over an estimated 6-month period. Assume the normal fee is $95 per session. You would agree to provide 6 months' worth of therapy for $2,280 (24 sessions × $95). The number of sessions would be estimated by the therapist with the understanding that the actual number of sessions might vary a little at the client's discretion. In the current example, the $2,280 fee would cover 20 to 28 visits. If fewer than 20 visits occurred, a rebate would be given. Visits beyond 28 would be charged at your regular fee. At the end of the 6-month period, a new treatment plan would be formulated, if necessary, with a new negotiation. Both the client's money and your investment are safeguarded within reasonable limits. The client has the advantage of combining predictable payments with the flexibility of some bonus visits if needed.

A disadvantage of this plan is that it is complicated. It requires a fair amount of education of your clients, because it is different. This raises an important point. No matter what fee plan you choose, *educate your clients up front.* If, out of your own anxiety over money, you fail to confront payment issues, you create the possibility of (1) damaging your therapy relationship and (2) getting involved in legal actions that are unpleasant at best. The impetus for a large number of *malpractice* actions is an attempt by a therapist to collect unpaid fees.

For my own practice, I chose to modify this plan, using a prepayment method. After an assessment of client needs, a treatment plan is proposed, perhaps 24 sessions over a 6-month period. The client can prepay the full amount in exchange for a 10% discount. Extra sessions, lengthy (over 10 minutes) phone consultations, testing, and other services are billed separately. If treatment ends for any reason prior to the planned number of sessions, unused sessions are refunded at the discounted rate. At the end of 6 months, treatment needs are reevaluated, and, if appropriate, an additional treatment contract is negotiated. Thus far, only one of my clients has opted for this plan. However, other therapists report more of their clients have elected this option.

Credit Cards

Whatever plans you use, accept credit cards. A certain number of clients will use them and deal with the bank about payments. This leaves you doing what you do best and the bank working within its area of expertise.

It is relatively easy to set up this program. Just call a bank. Any bank is willing to walk you through the steps because they want your business. However, do shop around. The bank makes its money by charging you a percentage of the credit card billings. This percentage varies from bank to bank. It also varies on the basis of how much is charged through your office. The more that is charged, the lower the interest charge is. In the program we use at the Manassas Group, the interest charge varies between 2% and 3%, depending on volume. This is an expense, but consider it the cost of collecting some fees at the time of visit that may otherwise turn into bad debts. The longer the period of time between providing the service and when payment is expected, the higher the rate of default on payments.

One therapist told me that accepting credit cards bothered her. She was concerned that doing so would encourage irresponsible use of credit, a growing problem in our society. However, our concern for clients should not lead us to make decisions for them. That is disempowering, no matter how good our intentions may be. We can offer choices and help clients to think through the consequences of those choices when appropriate, but we overstep our bounds when we make the decisions for them.

Bank Plans

One possibility is to explore making arrangements with a local bank for lower-interest loans for clients. The bank would offer the discount based on expected volume. The disadvantage is that it is hard to get banks interested. It is hard for them to predict volume, and it is an unsecured loan. In addition, from their perspective, the potential borrowers may be seen as mentally unstable. I believe that, as we move away from the medical model and therapy becomes more normalized, this will be less of a problem. For now, however, it is a problem, as the bank I consulted about this plan confirmed. While this plan may not currently have widespread applicability, its potential may grow over the years. A local bank has recently begun working on a reduced loan rate plan with a local plastic surgeon.

Insurance

I do still work with insurance reimbursement. About one-third of my clients still elect to use their health insurance. I do not chase them away. My approach is to educate clients about their alternatives, including the benefits of not using insurance reimbursement. Then we work together to help them decide which choices are best for their situation.

Lost Business. Sometimes therapists ask me whether I lose business because I am not on managed care panels. In their experience, potential clients phone in but decline to schedule once they learn a therapist is not on their panel. I do lose a few clients this way. It does not worry me. First, I am keeping a full schedule. Second, the people who do schedule seem committed to our work, making it more emotionally rewarding for me. In my experience, people who focus heavily on the cost of therapy often do not make much change regardless of the financial arrangements we make. Third, the economic range of my clients, which has always been broad, has not changed since I made these changes in my business practices. My practice has not come to focus just on the "carriage trade."

One participant in our seminars noted that his approach to this problem has been to invite reluctant callers in for a free "get acquainted" interview. He has found that, once people get to know him, they often can work out a mutually agreeable financial arrangement. Remember that our challenge is not just to fill our hours. Anyone can do that. Our challenge is to fill our hours in a profitable manner, both financially and emotionally.

PRESENTING YOURSELF TO YOUR COMMUNITY

Remember that no one responds to uninterpreted reality, including you. We can respond only to our *perceptions* of reality. Your image is the way you are perceived by your community. Determine what image you want to establish in your community. After you decide how you would like your community to see you, consider the factors that will combine to create such a public image. These factors will affect how you organize and locate your practice. Of course, it is important to be sure that the image you project is congruent with your actual identity. Incongruence between image and identity can create serious ethical and business problems when we do our marketing.

When the people in your community do not know you well, they will infer much from the few outward signs you offer: office location, parking, facilities, telephone and staff contacts, yellow page ads, and brochures. Placing your office in a well-known office park, surrounded by other professionals, sends one message. Having your office in your home sends another. Consider which will appeal to your potential clientele. Get into their heads. Which location suggests that you are serious about doing business? Which is more likely to lead people to confuse therapy with friendship? Which is more likely to place you at risk for accusations of unprofessional behavior?

Consider your office staff. As I mentioned, the Manassas Group favors using only high-quality office staff. We believe that having high-quality people sends a message of professionalism to the community. The feedback from our community suggests that they agree and value that aspect of our practice. Perhaps you respond: "Sure, but you can afford it. There are 15 of you." True. Yet, once there were only 2 of us, and we still had a full-time secretary/receptionist. We would not have considered doing business without her. Just her ability to make people feel comfortable during initial phone calls drew more than enough business to pay her salary. In addition, she saved us countless hours by handling all the paperwork, correspondence, scheduling, and fee collection in the most efficient way possible. She was a professional and extremely good at what she did. While she was doing what she did best, we were doing what we did best — doing the therapy that generated the fees that paid her salary and kept our practice open. Her salary was not so much an expense as it was an investment.

Further, consider the advantages of having a live person who is actively interested in your practice answering your phone. This can mean a lot to a potential client who may have taken days to gather the courage to call you. It also sends potential clients a message that you care enough about them to have a live, friendly person waiting for them when they call.

Because we have not had training in business of practice skills, we have underestimated the impact of these issues. If we are serious about conducting a private pay practice in these competitive times, then we must communicate that seriousness to potential clients. Our market niche is quality service. A high-quality office staff and a pleasant office send messages about commitment to quality that words alone cannot match.

YOUR OFFICE POLICIES

You need to make certain decisions about how you want to provide services. Unless you make well-considered conscious choices, you will be pressured into making some decisions that may not be the best.

For example, what hours will you be available? In my case, for example, as I was establishing a new practice that focused on children and families, I experienced a great deal of pressure to see people in the evenings. I did not want to. I had three children at home who needed a full-time father. How could I justify telling parents to spend more time with their children when I was not doing it myself? How could I justify my absence to my children? Furthermore, my own biological rhythms are such that I need a certain amount of downtime, best found in the evening. Therefore, I passed up some business, but the right schedule worked to my long-term advantage. People understood my reasons. Many clients told me that they admired my willingness to set limits and appreciated my commitment to my family. When my children started school, and the bus began picking them up at 7:00 A.M., I did begin to see some early morning clients.

What will your policies be with regard to cancellations? Under what conditions will you charge for cancelled sessions? What kind of message does your policy send about how much you value your time and service? A reasonable policy (at least I think so, which is why I use it) is to charge for failure to give at least 24 hours' notice of cancellation. I "forgive" the first such occurrence, with a restatement of the policy to the client. Very few clients miss more than once. If school is closed due to snow (or if I cannot get to my office due to snow), charges are not made. Unless the client goes to the doctor, illness is not excused. Nor is car trouble. I expect people to make some effort to get to appointments. This lets them know that I value our time and that effort is a necessary part of the process. If you are too lax, thinking that you are doing your clients a favor, you may find that you have many "no-shows."

BUSINESS ORGANIZATION

Do you want to be on your own, or do you want to affiliate with others? Each option has its advantages.

Many in our profession treasure solo practice. Pressure by managed care to move into group practices is one of the factors that distressed many therapists. Loss of autonomy is a major issue. We want to be able to practice as our individual conscience dictates and our personality prefers. It is not surprising that a profession designed to help people establish their individuality would consist of a lot of individualists.

However, there are disadvantages to solo practice, as well. Depending on your social needs, it can be extremely lonely. That loneliness could contribute to your becoming vulnerable to a blurring of boundaries between therapy and friendship. Practicing alone also makes it more difficult, though not impossible, to seek out consultation for those tough clinical issues. A group offers the opportunity for more capital, both financial and intellectual. The intellectual capital is important because, as you try to think through all the complexities of establishing a managed care free practice, having colleagues will help. The financial capital that a group can supply is clearly an advantage.

Yet, belonging to a group may interfere with your autonomy. Confronting these issues at the Manassas Group led us to evolve a model that serves both needs. Perhaps it will appeal to you. In 1980, my partner, Lou, and I set up shop. Within a few years, other therapists began to ask to join us. We did the natural thing. We hired them. At first we were all happy. That did not last. The superior-versus-subordinate aspect of employment did not suit the fact that we were professional peers. Our relationships began to suffer.

Today, each therapist in the Manassas Group is in business for himself/herself. Each person decides how much to work, what to charge, what services to deliver, how to deliver them, and so on. Lou and I own a corporation that provides services and facilities to the therapists for a percentage of billings. The corporation provides office space, telephones, secretary and receptionist services, basic office supplies, etc. We manage the day-to-day operation in exchange for profits we make from that percentage. Those profits also recognize the capital we have at risk.

For our group, this arrangement has many advantages: (1) Therapist autonomy is maximized within a group atmosphere, (2) colleagues are conveniently located nearby for social contact and consultation, (3) we can combine our resources to do group marketing as the group sees fit, and (4) the costs of doing business are reduced because of economies of scale.

CAPITAL

Statistics tell us that the vast majority of new businesses fail within a few years of start-up. The major reason is that the business is undercapitalized. The practice of therapy has long been seen as a low capital operation. Relatively speaking, this is true. Running a therapy practice requires less capital than, say, building cars or even running a hardware store. However, it does require some capital. If you do not plan adequately, you will be out of business. Therefore, as you make your business plan (and your marketing plan [see Chapter 8]), give thought to how much money you will need to get started and to keep going until your cash flow can meet your business expenses and personal financial needs.

If you are making a transition, rather than starting a practice from scratch, consider what costs you will incur. For example, you initially may lose some income, as I did, by not working with managed care. Or you may need to make some investments in new brochures and other marketing tools. You may decide to upgrade your office equipment and furniture. Or you may decide the value of secretarial help is worth the investment.

How will you fund these capital needs? First, consider your resources, which include your current income, savings, and investments. Do a financial statement. Any bank can give you a form that will ask the right questions. What is your net worth? Which of the assets that create that net worth do you dare access for this venture? Which assets would you decide are untouchable? Second, what can you borrow? People take out loans to fund business ventures all the time. All of this, of course, is part of the risk of being an entrepreneur. It is less risky if you have a well-thought-out plan. Also, having sufficient capital, even if it means taking the risk of borrowing, reduces your long-term risk because you are giving yourself a serious chance at success.

FURTHER TRAINING

As you consider making a transition to private pay based therapy, you may find that you want to obtain further training. There may be certain traditional services about which you want to learn more. Or you may be interested in some of the diversifications available but need more training. Get it.

You must be willing to invest enough time and money in your business. Remember that you are the primary tool of this business. Good tools are the backbone of a successful business. Give yourself permission to get enough training to feel comfortable and competent in delivering high-quality services.

SUMMARY

You have now answered many of the questions necessary to create a sound business plan, the foundation for your practice (fill in Box 7.6). You have developed a concrete vision of your future and developed ways to get there.

Now it is time to go public. Chapter 8 will show you how.

BOX 7.6. Writing a Business Plan

A business plan is like a good theory of therapy. It guides but does not dictate decision making. This outline will help you organize your thinking as you approach your new endeavors. Take as much time as you need to complete your responses.

1. What business are you in? What services do you or will you provide?

   _____

   _____

   _____

   _____

   _____

2. Write a mission statement (1–3 sentences)

   _____

   _____

   _____

3. Who is your competition?

   _____

   _____

   _____

   _____

4. What advantages do you offer over your competition? How can you work together?

   _____

   _____

   (*cont.*)

(continued from previous page)

_____

_____

_____

5. What advantages do your competitors have over you?

_____

_____

_____

_____

_____

_____

6. Pricing
   a. What are the costs of running your practice?
      (That information is in Box 7.5.)   _____
   b. What is your annual net income goal?   _____
      (If you set a goal, you have a chance to
      achieve it.)
   c. What is the range of your competitors' fees?   _____
   d. How many billable hours do you have available? _____
   e. Given this information, what do you plan to
      charge for your various services?

                        Description   *Fee*
         Service A: _____   _____
         Service B: _____   _____
         Service C: _____   _____
         Service D: _____   _____

7. What payment policies will you have in force?

_____

_____

_____

_____

_____

(cont.)

(continued from previous page)

8. Factors that establish your identity with the public
   a. Office location _____
   b. Available parking_____
   c. Telephone arrangements _____
   d. Office staff _____

9. Office policies
   a. Hours you are available _____
   b. Your access for emergencies _____
   c. Cancellation policies _____

10. What kind of business structure will you use?
   _____ Solo practice   _____ Partnership
   _____ Group practice _____ Institutional
   _____ Other (describe: _____
   _____)

11. How will you fund your business? What resources can you call on?

   _____

   _____

   _____

   _____

   _____

   _____

12. What additional training would be helpful, either in acquiring new skills or in boosting your self-confidence?

   _____

   _____

   _____

   _____

   _____

Chapter 8

How to Market Traditional Services

Now that you have developed a business plan, let's go find some business. This means marketing. Recall our definition of marketing. It is a two-step process of education. First, you learn what your potential clients want or need. Second, you find ways to let them know you have services that speak to those wants and needs. Having done one or more of the free market studies suggested in Chapter 6, you have already begun marketing. What this chapter does is to show you how to do the second part of marketing—finding and educating potential clients. Then we will help you to come up with a marketing plan of your own.

Historically, most therapists have relied on gatekeepers to send referrals. You will see that this continues to be an important element of marketing, though with some new touches. However, if we were to rely *solely* on gatekeepers, we would be keeping ourselves in a dependent relationship. Therefore, as we create a marketing plan, we will include plans for effective connections with gatekeepers, but we will pay a lot more attention to strategies for going directly to the public.

THE SIX QUESTIONS OF MARKETING

By answering six questions (see Box 8.1), you can determine how to market your services. There are many ways to answer these questions. That is part of the fun of marketing.

As mentioned a number of times, we have historically felt uncomfortable about marketing. Only part of our reluctance in this area was

---

BOX 8.1. The Six Questions of Marketing

1. What services will you provide?
2. Who are your potential candidates for each service?
3. Where can you find them?
4. What value does your service have for them?
5. How can you communicate this value to them in terms they will understand?
6. How can you establish with potential clients that you are a credible source of the service?

---

based on ethical concerns. The other factor was a lack of skill that was painfully obvious whenever we made attempts to market. The mistake most of us made was to *begin* our marketing plans by asking the fifth question in this six-question series. We cannot competently answer question 5 until we answer the preceding questions. No wonder we felt that this stuff was beyond us! You will see that, as you answer these questions in order, your ability to create a competent marketing plan will be up to the task.

1. What Services Will You Provide?

You have already answered this question. In your business plan, you identified the services that you plan to provide. Different services that you offer require different answers to each of the next five questions.

2. Who Are Your Potential Candidates for Each Service?

Responding to this question builds a picture of the people with whom you want to work. Who *are* the people who are candidates for the particular service you want to provide? It is not everyone in the world. As you define your candidates, it will become increasingly easy to figure out how to reach them with your message. You can identify them by thinking through the series of questions listed in Box 8.2.

What geographical area will you mainly serve? Most Manassas Group clients come from within the Roanoke Valley, a metropolitan area of about one-quarter of a million people. However, since Roanoke is the largest city within southwestern Virginia, some people travel up to 80 miles, one

---

**BOX 8.2. General Questions to Identify
Your Potential Clients**

1. What geographical area will you mainly serve?
2. What income levels will you mainly serve?
3. What age groups do you want to serve?
4. What are the life roles of people who could use your services?
5. What special populations are of interest to you?

---

way, to see us. If your practice is in Manhattan, you probably serve a smaller geographical area.

What is the income level of the people you want to see? One of the traditional mistakes of therapists considering a private pay practice is to overestimate how high a family's income must be to afford to pay out of pocket. Of course, there is a lower limit, not counting whatever pro bono work you may choose to do. Maslow's pyramid accurately predicts that people at the lower end of the economic scale choose food and shelter over therapy. By choosing to be in private practice, you have in effect decided that the large majority of your clientele will not come from the bottom rung of the economic ladder.

Certainly, the higher the family income, the easier it is for people to decide to purchase therapy services, just as it is easier for them to make any other purchase. How you price your services and what payment policies you develop will also have an impact on who will have financial access to you.

Beyond those constraints, the lower limit of family income will depend on where therapy fits within the family's priorities. If it is a high priority, most people will find the money. If therapy is seen as fluff or shameful, you will be lucky if your services come in somewhere below dog food. Where therapy fits within the family's priorities will depend, in large part, on how well we communicate about the value of our services.

Now locate the neighborhoods within the geographical area you defined earlier that have a predominance of people within your economic parameters. This does not mean you will not accept referrals from other areas. All that you are doing is trying to build a picture within your own mind of your potential clientele.

What age groups do you want to serve? What age groups are you *trained* to serve? You need both training and desire to do a good job. Do you want to work just with adults? Are children's issues the ones that make your eyes light up? What about adolescents and the elderly?

What are the life roles of people who could use your services? For example, are they parents, students, executives, married, single, or in the sandwich generation? This may be one of the most important questions to answer because life roles dictate the life issues people are facing and that may be causing them trouble.

What special populations are of interest to you? In Chapter 6, for example, mention was made of sex offenders, a special population whose demographics may cut across many of the classifications identified so far.

Notice that, as you answer each of these general questions, the picture of your clientele begins to come into better focus. You realize that you know more than you may have thought, once you know what questions to answer. It is a lot like therapy. The hardest part is knowing the right questions to ask. As your picture's clarity improves, the chances of successful communication between you and potential clients improve as well.

So far we have looked at general questions. Now let's get a bit more specific by considering the particular services that you want to provide, either entry-level or long-range services. Let's use an example. Suppose the story about the college food manager cited in Chapter 6 grabbed your attention. This was the fellow who hid the college newspapers when the cafeteria's food got a bad review. You might decide that your interests and expertise converge in the area of helping people to build decision-making skills under pressure. Within the limits already established, who are candidates for your service?

Executives come to mind. Executives must make decisions all the time. In addition, young lawyers, young physicians, young architects, and other young professionals all must make decisions quickly, but their relative inexperience is likely to make them quite uneasy. Imagine a group of young executives, lawyers, doctors, therapists, and dentists telling stories, offering support, and seeing that they share similar pressures. On second thought, never mind imagining it—make it happen! Also, young parents come to mind. Many young mothers and fathers, overwhelmed by the demands of childrearing, become terrified about some of their decision making, and they, too, need our help.

For practice, let's consider another example from Chapter 6: Some people are afraid to fly. Suppose you wanted to expand this service to helping people when anxiety got in the way of normal daily activities. Candidates for your service would include people who avoided flying because of fear, people who avoided the dentist out of fear, people afraid to give public talks or performances, people afraid to drive, and people afraid to leave their homes.

3. Where Can You Find Potential Clients?

Now that you have a picture of what your candidates look like, you want to figure out more specifically where to find them. To understand this process, imagine a funnel. The wide part of the funnel represents your entire community. The narrow part of the funnel is where your candidates come together. They may in fact hang out together at certain times, or they may be likely to pass through certain domains (professional offices, work sites, recreational facilities, clubs, etc.) via shared experiences.

For example, your definition of young decision makers as potential clients helps you to figure out where the narrow part of the funnel is. Companies with a large number of white-collar jobs are likely to have a collection of new executives. Such companies often have training programs for young executives, which your program might supplement. Large law firms, medical practices, architectural firms, and the like may well be part of the narrow part of the funnel. They too are interested in the development of their new professionals.

Where do young parents hang out? Pediatricians' offices, OB/GYN offices, churches, and PTA gatherings are some possibilities that come to mind. If you focus on physicians, remember to differentiate your services from mental health work. Otherwise, the physicians will forget that referrals to you for your services will not count against their financial reimbursements from HMOs.

What about people whose anxiety gets in the way of living? Travel agents may have access to spouses of people who are afraid to fly ("I'd like to fly to Phoenix, but my wife is too afraid—what are the rail connections like?"). Dentists have had contact with people too fearful to keep appointments or with parents of children whose fear makes dental work impossible. (One of my first long-term play therapy clients was a girl too fearful to get the dental services she needed. I worked with that family on and off for years on a broad range of issues.) Toastmasters is an organization that helps people learn how to do public talks or presentations. Anxiety is a common barrier to making the transition from talking at Toastmasters to talking in public. People who are afraid to drive may be reacting to the experience of an automobile accident. Such people pass through emergency rooms, lawyers' offices, and auto insurance agencies. People afraid to go out of their home still read the newspaper.

Each of these ideas represents the narrow part of a funnel. Consider the potential candidates for the services *you* want to provide. Where are the narrow parts of the funnel for them? During our seminars, we do an exercise in which we take examples through these six marketing questions. What usually happens is that it is not hard to identify a service. When we get to the part about defining candidates, the obvious answer is given first. Then comes silence. I wait. Before long, participants begin to have lots of additional ideas about who candidates for the service in question can be. A similar process happens when participants begin to identify the narrow parts of the funnel. At first, the ideas about where to find candidates come slowly. Then a dam bursts and suddenly many ideas pour forth. Therefore, as you try to answer these questions for your services, expect a stuck point. Don't quit. More ideas will come, especially if you brainstorm with other people.

For example, in one seminar, the service under question was helping singles build skills to establish successful, enduring relationships with significant others. When I asked where single individuals typically hang out, the first response was "at work," a good answer. Then there was silence for a brief time as people considered other possibilities. Within a minute, many additional good answers were given: "singles" apartments, the library, laundry rooms and laundromats, bookstores, grocery stores, churches, health clubs, bars, college facilities, and hair salons.

4. What Value Does Your Service Have for Potential Clients?

Now the task is to articulate the value your service has to the candidate. Here the focus is on the service, not you. We will get to you later. As we have discussed, the value will be in the benefits that clients derive from your services, not in the features (methods) of those services. Therefore, as you answer this question, focus on the *anticipated results*. That is what will be of interest to your potential clients.

It is essential to make the case that the service provided is both useful and valuable to potential clients. Otherwise, they have no reason to give you their money. Consider how you spend money. If you go browsing to consider buying your first computer, you have to be convinced that you even need or could use a computer. Its value to you must be established. Once that happens, you will want to know why one computer serves your needs better than another. If your salesperson responds to either of these issues with "Gee. I don't know," are you likely to buy? Suppose, on the other hand, the salesperson listens carefully and then helps to establish how a computer might have benefits for you and your goals. Then the salesperson helps you to differentiate good candidates from bad. Now what happens to your chances of buying?

If you want to market services to improve decision-making skills under pressure, you must clearly demonstrate their value. Why would people want help with decision-making skills? There are lots of reasons. Young executives and young professionals could get a competitive boost over others in their field. They would be less likely to make "rookie" mistakes if they could allow their training to guide them, rather than their anxiety. Better performance could be emotionally and financially rewarding. Young parents would feel more confident in their skills. Relationships with children would be improved. Episodes of abuse would be fewer. These are all good results that people would value.

With regard to anxiety reduction services, the value could also be high. People would be able to fly, get dental care, speak in public, drive and see their children's school plays instead of being imprisoned in their own home. These are tremendous values.

Why would someone seek therapy for academic underachievement? A number of psychological issues can impair achievement. Dealing with those issues can sometimes remove the impairment. A participant in our first seminar shared the following:

> He was a college freshman — for the third time. His parents had spent $51,000 on his college education, only to see very little education. His older siblings had achievement patterns more consistent with the parents' professional lifestyle. Why did the third one progress so little? Was this young man simply goofing off? His visible despair did not support that conclusion. What about drugs or alcohol abuse? Again, that did not fit the picture. Our seminar participant gave the client a psychological evaluation, including an IQ test. He scored in the mid-80s. He was never going to find college to be a place of success.
>
> While in some ways the IQ test results were not good news, there was considerable relief in having an answer. This young man could now focus his energies in areas that could lead to success for him. He no longer had to follow the examples set by his older siblings. His parents loved him dearly and were relieved to see his stress evaporate. These personal outcomes made the service highly valuable to all concerned.
>
> In addition, there was the money. The psychological evaluation cost $500. Too bad it did not happen before the parents spent $51,000 on college. The financial return here is pretty clear.

When answering the question about what value your services have, be prepared to meet objections. Think through the arguments *against* your particular services. For example, why shouldn't people "just forget" about past traumas? Why shouldn't underachieving students simply be made to work harder? Why shouldn't young professionals already know how to handle pressure?

You already have experience in overcoming objections. Nearly everyone you see has demonstrated resistance of one kind or another during therapy. As you have responded to that resistance, you have at times articulated how the value of what you are asking clients to do exceeds the cost to them of time, money, effort, and fear. Call on these experiences and memories as you articulate the answers to the objections that people may raise about your services.

Test your ideas by explaining them to friends and colleagues who like you too much to just be polite. Explaining ideas to others forces us to hear ourselves in different ways. Considering objections in advance might enable you to find a fatal flaw in a service that initially sounded good. Or perhaps the flaw can be corrected with a bit of retooling. It is better that you find the flaws and remove them than to have potential clients find them and then avoid you.

5. How Can You Communicate About the Value of Your Service?

Having established in your own mind the value of the service to the people you consider as candidates for it, you are in a position to figure out how to go about sending the message.

There are a number of marketing tools that various small businesses use in educating the public, or selected target audiences, about goods and services. Remember that people can make informed decisions only if we present them with relevant information. However, we need to present this information in a professional manner. Professionalism means that we do not make claims we cannot back up or promises we cannot keep. However, maintaining a professional stance does not mean that we have to under-promise. Underpromising also fails to give accurate information. Nor does it mean we cannot be creative in our educational efforts. Today, boringly presented messages do not get received. They get ignored.

Professionalism also means that we do not pretend to be the only ones with the answer. We do not take the position that our methods are superior to everyone else's. Not only is that likely to exceed the data that justifies our services, it is bad business. Marketing that relies on tearing others down is rarely effective. Talk about what you can really do and the outcomes people can really expect. The truth holds more than enough value to lead most people to your door.

Finally, professionalism means that we do not manipulate people's emotions. I fear that some hospital ads I saw recently have begun to violate that particular ethic. We should not scare people into seeing us, or "guilt" people into seeing us, or intimidate them. We should simply demonstrate that we bring understanding and guidance to a problem that bothers them. We should help those affected to create an honest vision of what solving that problem would look like, and what it might accomplish.

Guerrilla Marketing (1993) by Jay Conrad Levinson offers a wealth of marketing tools and strategies. Levinson's target audience is small business owners like us rather than megacorporations. His intention is to offer creative and inexpensive marketing tools to businesses small enough to be flexible and nimble. Many of the strategies he presents can be made appropriate to professional endeavors, while some cannot. What follows is a *partial* list of possible marketing tools that Levinson offers in his book. (I left out searchlights, e.g., not being creative enough to find a professional way to use them. Perhaps you will find a way. If so, feel free to add them back.)

A Sampling of Marketing Tools

Canvassing	Outdoor signs
Personal letters	Yellow pages ads
"Guerrilla" business cards	Newspaper ads
(cards that describe your	Magazine ads
service, not just provide your	Radio/TV ads
name)	Direct mail
Telephone marketing	Imprinted pens and pencils
Circulars and brochures	Seminars and demonstrations
Signs on bulletin boards	Sponsorship of events
Classified ads	Exhibits at trade shows

Levinson goes on to present a wealth of information to fledgling marketers like us. In addition to outlining basic marketing, his book will walk you through many of the technical ins and outs. He will help you to evaluate the pros and cons of newspaper ads versus magazine ads versus radio ads versus direct mail. He will show you how to save money on whatever marketing tools you choose. What follows is some information that I particularly wanted to bring to your attention.

First, plan to spend some money. It does not have to be a huge sum. In fact, Levinson prides himself on helping people to figure out inexpensive ways to market. However, you will need to spend something. Again, remember that you are in business. Some of the money you make is profit. Take it home. Some of the money you make *must* be put back into the business as an investment. This is the same principle that farmers follow, among whom "eating your seed corn" is a sure sign of folly (quickly followed by the demise of the farm). Levinson argues that part of a good marketing program is an adequate marketing budget. He suggests that you specify a given "percentage of sales" that will be available for continual marketing.

Your campaign needs to *make* your candidates familiar with you and *keep* them familiar with you. Levinson presents two interesting facts that tell why both requirements are important. He notes that Americans are exposed to 2,700 marketing messages a day. They might be forgiven for missing one or two. You do not want them to miss your message.

Yet, even if they see your message today, it may get pushed out of their mind by tomorrow's onslaught of messages. Periodic repetition increases the chance that your message will be seen *and* remembered. To illustrate this point, Levinson reports a study on people's *memory* of newspaper ads. A weekly newspaper ad was run for 13 weeks. At the end of that time, 63% of readers recalled seeing the ad. One month later, only 32% recalled it. Two weeks after that, 21% remembered it. If you market to the public, you have to find a way to keep your name in front of them or your name will soon be replaced by someone else's name. Your message may not be relevant to someone today, whereas a month from now, it might be. If your message shows up periodically, your target audience will take greater notice of your message over time, which is exactly what you want. Levinson summarizes the issue as follows: "Consistency equates with familiarity. Familiarity equates with confidence. And confidence equates with sales" (p. 27).

Levinson points out that the most frequent fatal error of would-be marketers is to implement a plan and then give up on it too quickly. His advice is to work out your doubts in advance by doing your homework. This fits well for people like us, with heavy academic backgrounds. We know how to do our homework. In this case, homework means taking time to create a program that you have reason to believe will be successful. It means checking it out; trouble-shooting it with friends, family, and maybe clients. Do not begin it until you have reasonable confidence in what you have put together.

Once you have that confidence, give your program enough time to work. Levinson says that marketing programs usually do not even *begin* to show results before 60 days. Sometimes they take up to a year. Without sufficient appreciation of reasonable expectations, many of us have "tried" a marketing strategy only to quit too soon. We then come to believe that we do not know how to market. In reality, we might know how to market—but not know how to wait.

I was admittedly one of those impatient marketers. Some years ago, Lou and I decided to hold some seminars for the public to increase our visibility. I had developed a presentation on "Power in the Family" that had already been well received at a large community gathering. It seemed like a natural to me, so we ran an ad in the newspaper. That's right—we ran *an* ad. The turnout was zero. We did not begin to invest enough time (or money) in this endeavor to give it even a long shot at success. That is not a mistake I will repeat.

6. How Can You Establish Your Credibility?

You need to help people see you as a credible source of the service that you are marketing. It does no good to convince someone that the service is valuable if they do not recognize that you are a good provider of that service. How can you present yourself so that people will have confidence in you?

Like it or not, repetition will accomplish some of this aim. People tend to forget where they obtain information. Once your name becomes familiar in the community, people will assume you must have some credibility or you would not have been around so long. Perhaps there is some truth to that.

Your credentials can help some, though perhaps less than we might like to believe. Recall our yellow pages examples and the low impact of board certification. However, establishing yourself through your marketing as a trained, licensed behavioral scientist does serve to differentiate you from the unqualified opportunists.

Offering services that speak to an urgent concern that people have helps to establish credibility. "Someone knows what I need!" is the common response. Communicating intelligently about the service also establishes credibility. However, this must be done in everyday language, not jargon. You are not trying to draw in your graduate professors for treatment, but rather those people you have defined as likely candidates for your service. It is your responsibility to show that you know your field well enough to present it clearly to ordinary people with problems.

Another method of establishing credibility in the eyes of the public is through a good public relations campaign. Public relations may be defined as getting attention from the media without paying money for it, though you will spend effort and time. The benefit you can achieve is to have people in your community begin to see you as an expert in dealing with certain problems of urgent concern to them.

The effort and time you spend will be in drawing the attention of reporters and other media gatekeepers. Like our candidates for services, reporters are people with problems. Their chief occupational problem is to come up with interesting material to fill their papers and broadcasts everyday. You can help them solve that problem. The public is interested, fascinated perhaps, by the things that you and I deal with daily. Therefore, you have something—information, data, theories, opinions—that the reporter can use. As you provide this information, you demonstrate your expertise, the public becomes familiar with your name, and the reporter gets a story. Everybody benefits.

How do you begin? One approach would be to hire a public relations professional to help you gain access to the media. The Virginia Academy of Clinical Psychologists hired a PR consultant to help with the Virginia Marketing Project and found her to be both professional and helpful, although her role for us focused more on relating to the business community than the media. A PR consultant could provide you with personalized ways to gain access to the media using relationships she probably already has.

Of course, there is an expense involved here. You can avoid this expense by doing your own PR program, if you are willing to do your homework. Again, doing homework is our forte. My mother, Bonnie Ackley, was a public relations professional for 25 years and shared the following tips for us to use:

• First, you must respect the media, its people and its purposes. Many people blame the media for our society's ills, and it must take its share of the blame, but not a disproportionate amount. All professions have their share of bad apples. When they are in the media, they are very public. For the most part, though, news professionals have ethical standards that they value, just as other professionals do. Reporters need to report about what is happening that affects all of us, and if you help them report the news accurately and fairly, they will welcome you. If you do not respect the media, it will show.

• Don't ever tell a reporter you have a great story you want published. Tell him you have an idea that may be interesting to him. He is not going to want you to write his story. He needs to control what is written. Telling him you have an idea that may be interesting communicates that you and the reporter can cooperate in getting the story out accurately.

• Don't call a reporter anytime close to press or air time to present an idea. He's busy. Call him after the presses start rolling or after the news show, when he has time to listen to you. Don't call on Mondays. Newsrooms are scrambling to catch up on the weekend happenings.

• Find out who is the right person to contact: the business editor, the family page editor, the news director at the radio or TV station, or the feature writer on a local magazine. Get the name right.

• Many times, it is best to present your idea for a story in writing. Wait for a response. Don't call to ask why you have not had an answer or when the story will run. Reporters operate on their timetable, not yours. It is possible, however, to write a follow-up letter that asks if there is further information needed.

• You and your associates can invite the media (get the right names on the invitations) to a breakfast in which you give them your viewpoints on topics of interest today, such as managed care, violence in the workplace, the new role of the therapist in America, or whatever topic you believe will intrigue the reporters. Serve a light breakfast. Respect your guests' time restrictions and keep the meeting short. Have your best spokesperson make the presentation.

• Write to the program directors of your local radio and television stations, offering to be interviewed when a crisis has occurred or when a troublesome situation is developing in the community. Give your credentials.

• Find out when the local newspaper will run its annual section on health and submit an article to the editor. Discuss common family problems such as teen problems or stepparenting, school difficulties, or any other subject that will interest everyone. Stay away from dealing with runaway daughters or kleptomaniac grandmothers in the house. These are too scary, feeding the notion that only the terribly strange and disturbed consult you. Let your article demonstrate how therapists can help ordinary people solve ordinary problems. In that vein, write in English, not jargon.

Many of us struggle with "microphone and camera anxiety," which may keep us from following up on these suggestions. *Of course* you are nervous if this is new to you. However, there are ways to make the anxiety manageable:

• Information reduces anxiety. If a reporter calls you for a story, learn about what she wants from you, how much time she needs, when her deadline is, and her goal for the story.

• Preparation reduces anxiety. Figure out what you want to say. Reduce it in your mind to two or three main points. Figure out how to make your points in everyday language. Review your ideas before the interview with someone whose opinion you respect. If the reporter throws you a curve, acknowledge her question but politely work your way back to the points *you* want to make.

• Wearing the right clothes reduces anxiety. Dressing in a manner that reflects your professional identity will help your sense of confidence.

• Relaxation exercises reduce your anxiety. Use the method of your choice. My favorite is hypnosis. Before any public speaking or media presentation that I anticipate will elevate my anxiety significantly, my preparation includes taking myself into a trance by focusing on a peaceful experience. Within the trance, I recall successful presentations and interviews in the past. Then, I rehearse for the upcoming event. This formula has been extremely helpful to me in calling on my resources in the actual event.

Want more information? Read Marcia Yudkin's book *Six Steps to Free Publicity* (1994).

Measuring results. There is one more step to a marketing program, namely, measuring its results. This is a step that therapists often skip. Foregoing this step is like typing on a word processor without a monitor: How can you tell if you have made a mistake?

Fortunately, evaluating the results of your various marketing efforts can be quite straightforward. As people come in your door, ask how they heard about you or your service. Continue or intensify the marketing methods people respond to and let the others go if they have had a fair shot. If no one comes in the door at all, it is not hard to evaluate the results.

YOUR MARKETING EFFORTS WITH GATEKEEPERS

Most of us who have a history of success in private practice have done a lot of networking with gatekeepers. The ideas we are considering can expand your success even with them. This is important because sometimes, when you market to the public, the narrow part of the funnel goes directly through a gatekeeper's office. What follows are some thoughts that go beyond the usual ways we have marketed through gatekeepers.

Special Note—Working with Physicians

Many therapists have worked hard to create and maintain referral relationships with physicians. Physicians have a history of being powerful gatekeepers for us. Given what is happening in the health care arena, the referral power of physicians is likely to decline. Certainly for physicians in capitated practices, the financial pressure *not to refer* will be high. The entire mind-set in a capitated system is to minimize service delivery. Within HMOs and vertically integrated health care monopolies, if a referral must be made, the pressure will be enormous to make that referral *in-house,* to therapists employed by the organization.

There is another issue that may lessen physicians' referral power. The dominant response by medicine to managed care, just like the dominant response of our own profession, has been to change practice patterns in deference to what managed care companies demand. Basically, this approach involves building a market on the basis of cost rather than on the basis of quality. *Breaking Free of Managed Care* is entirely about marketing on the basis of quality. If some significant segment of the medical community does not soon opt in a similar direction, the quality of medical care will suffer. This imminent debasement of their calling may well diminish physicians' credibility in the eyes of the public. People will be less likely to abide by suggestions of professionals with lowered credibility.

Thus, there are two reasons why physician referral power may be on the wane. If your practice has been largely based on physician referral, it is now time to widen your referral base.

A Modified Approach to Gatekeepers

Traditionally, we have looked for ways to educate gatekeepers about our services. We have delivered our messages over lunch, with brochures, and on the phone, saying thinks like, "I like to work with children," "I help depressed people," or "I do marital therapy." This approach has worked sort of well. But look at how each sentence focuses on us, not the referral source. We were essentially asking referral sources to solve our problem by sending us clients. This is one of many ways in which we have allowed ourselves to do business in a passive dependent manner. We now know that people respond to us best when we can solve *their* problem. Referral sources are no different from other people in that regard.

The key to successful networking with gatekeepers is similar to the one noted in our Chapter 5 discussion about presenting services to the public, as well as in our discussion in this chapter about reporters and public relations. Like everyone else, gatekeepers, usually professionals, are people with problems. The particular problems that interest us occur when their clients, patients, or customers ask them for assistance that they cannot give, or ask for a referral for that help. Gatekeepers want to respond in a way that strengthens and preserves their own relationship with their client, patient, or customer. Their own business well-being requires that they put that person in touch with an effective therapist who will make the client happy with the referral, strengthening the original relationship. You know this to be true from the times that you are the referring professional. You want things to go well for your client.

Gatekeepers respond positively to therapists who take problems off their hands. The way to network with them successfully, therefore, is to figure out what your target gatekeepers *worry* about—what keeps them up at night—and how you can take those problems off their hands. Then, they will see you as someone who has *value* to them.

Imagine the busy, harried attorney who has just received his umpteenth call from a divorced client furious with her ex-husband over yet another episode of tardy child-support payments. The attorney has run out of both patience and legal remedies for her, and he recognizes that what she and the whole family need most now is a therapeutic intervention that enables everyone to get on with life. Which therapist is the attorney going to refer this woman to—the one who has an ad full of credentials in the yellow pages or the one who took him to lunch last week to talk about helping people through the trauma of divorce? We must look at these issues from the gatekeeper's point of view, focusing on the benefits to him (i.e., a satisfied client no longer besieging him with phone calls) rather than on our specific methods of therapy.

Because you are now in the position of reorienting your practice, it would be easy and honest for you to approach various gatekeepers in the following way: "I am interested in expanding my services to the community. I would value your opinion about what services are most needed. Could we meet for lunch so that I could hear your ideas?" Most people feel flattered by such a request and are happy to spend the time. If you use this approach, be sure it is not a sham. Really listen. What you learn may be surprisingly helpful to you.

What this approach gives you is a fourth free (except for the cost of the lunch) market study. It allows you to hear about the needs of the community through the eyes of professionals in touch with many people in the community. Of course, no one's opinions are unbiased. In this case, that is an advantage. You will hear what makes each gatekeeper worry. It is these worries that motivate behavior, hopefully referral behavior.

As you listen to the gatekeeper's worries, let your imagination begin to work. You have begun to train your imagination by doing the earlier market study exercises. It has now begun to break free of the limits that the medical model had placed on it. As the gatekeeper talks, you will begin to see opportunities, ways that your favorite approaches to understanding and working with people can be applied to what worries the gatekeeper. As you listen carefully and ask probing questions (skills at which you are very good), you can begin to outline your preliminary ideas. Your gatekeeper is now participating with you in the creation of a new service. This participation will inspire a psychological sense of ownership, making the gatekeeper even more likely to refer to you.

Suppose your imagination just does not respond to the gatekeeper's concerns at that very moment. No problem! A respectful and relationship-building response might be: "That is an interesting problem. I can see why you're having so much trouble with it. I am not sure myself how to respond. What I would like to do is give it some thought and meet with you again when I have an idea. We could talk about it, and you could tell me what you think. Would 2 weeks from today be a good time?" By not having an instant answer, and admitting so, you have given the gatekeeper's problem credibility. By arranging another visit, you have done some relationship deepening. By setting a date for the visit, you make sure it will happen. Another free lunch wouldn't hurt either. Figure this into your financial plan. It is part of the cost of doing business.

Consultations

Another way to connect with gatekeepers is to create opportunities to consult with groups of potential referral sources. Such consultations will create referrals if you help gatekeepers solve problems that concern them.

Primary care physicians and the clergy have long been important referral sources to us because people frequently call on them for help with personal problems. We know that, as managed care grows, demands for mental health related services will grow even beyond their already high level. Similarly, with other avenues to helpful listening being closed by managed care, the clergy are likely to be even more besieged by their parishioners seeking personal counsel. This will create serious problems for physicians and the clergy, both in terms of time demands and in terms of being asked increasingly to handle situations for which they are not adequately prepared. Both of these problems will make them worry.

We can provide assistance. We can offer group consultation to physicians or to clergy around their difficult cases. You could meet with a group of four to eight professionals for, say, 2 hours a month, or with busy physicians, perhaps 1 hour twice a month. Group members would present cases for review, with both you and the group responding. This is a fairly standard group supervision format for us, but it may be a real treat for them. Encouraging group members to participate actively, rather than feeding the myth that you are the only one in the room with any competence in this area, would build their skills.

Your meeting could become a welcome refuge. I recently did a training exercise with a group of assistant principals for a school system. Part of our work involved dividing the principals into small groups to discuss their roles. This unavoidably led them to share difficulties they experience on the job. The overwhelming consensus was that this sharing was intensely meaningful. "This is the first time in 31 years I have had a chance to do this," one man declared.

While you want referrals, your task in these consultations is really to help your consultees provide better direct services. This will benefit those receiving services from your consultees because the providers' skills will be enhanced by your input. If you see this consultation *primarily* as a way to snarf referrals, your consultees will know it quickly and probably dismiss you. If you try to be genuinely helpful, they will value you. Many of the people they see are people who were unlikely to come to see you anyway. However, as the consultation process unfolds, your group members will unavoidably see, on their own, when they are in over their heads. When that happens, who will they refer to?

Through such a group consultation, you can help medical professionals provide short-term, symptom-based services. That is likely what they see as their usual role, anyway. However, this approach also gives you a nice chance to widen their understanding of therapy and its possibilities. You can help them see the value of ongoing trait-changing therapy, which they can then present to the individual seeking help. Who will get those referrals?

Finally, this consultation provides you an opportunity to educate these gatekeepers—whether medical or clerical—about your managed care free approach. Because this approach is so contrary to conventional wisdom, you will benefit from the repeated opportunities to demonstrate your value. It will help the gatekeepers understand, in an experiential way, that the people they refer to you will get what they pay for.

Given the comments made about the dying referral power of physicians, you may wonder about the wisdom of setting up the group consultation just discussed. But remember what we said earlier: There is a twist that may encourage physicians to refer to you *because of* your managed care free status. Your services will not count against the physician's capitation contract, since health insurance benefits are not used. Therefore, the physician *can* refer to you, but not to your managed care buddy, without having it go in the loss column at the end of the year. Physicians are unlikely to see this advantage without help from you. Most are trapped in the managed care mind-set, just as we have been. That mind-set can often blind people to certain opportunities.

While physician referral power may be declining, many other traditional gatekeepers still are available. Lawyers, judges, and school personnel, for example, are all still faced with problems for which you are a resource. As you broaden the kinds of services you deliver, you can be even more valuable. First, you will be able to speak to problems in living within the language spoken by those sources, making it easier for them to think of you.

Second, your potential referral sources will no longer have to try to make their clients fit into a mental health category. By reducing the shame barrier, you make it easier for gatekeepers to refer to you. Your potential referral sources will no longer have to imply that their client is "mentally ill" when they make the referral. Consider the burden lifted from your referral sources as they go about the delicate business of getting you and their client together. Many professionals do not make referrals simply because they do not want to deal with the reaction their clients might have to being sent to a shrink—namely, "You think I'm crazy?!" Remember, gatekeepers must protect their relationships with their clients. That usually means not insulting them.

One way to facilitate your referral sources' ability to refer to you is to develop some language they can use to explain your approach to their clients, patients, or customers. Since you are operating outside of conventional wisdom, your referral sources will need to be able to explain things in a rational, convincing manner. Help them to do so. You might also consider developing a brochure tailor-made for referral sources to give out at the time of referral that uses the desired language.

Contrast these two scenarios: (1) "I'd like to give you the name of an excellent therapist who comes highly recommended. . . . " [Client: "He thinks I'm crazy. I'm sorry I brought it up."] (2) "I know this guy who coaches people on this sort of thing all the time. He's really good. Maybe you could pick his brain. Of course, he costs money, but he's worth it. I've got his number here somewhere if you want to take it just in case." [Client: "Hey, this guy sounds good. I can't figure this thing out. It would be great if he could help me get a handle on it."] "Yeah, sure. Give me his number."

Finally, do not overlook employee assistance programs (EAPs) as a referral source for managed care free services. Of course, EAPs are operating out of the mental illness mind-set. However, *their urgent problem* is to save their client companies money. Anytime they can refer to you, the costs of service are not counted against them, any more than they are counted against those physicians in capitated contracts that we discussed earlier. EAPs are unlikely to think of this on their own. They will need your help.

Of course, when they make referrals, they have a responsibility to tell clients about the benefit program offered by their employer. There will be some clients who may be best served by using those programs. Others, however, will be better served by your approach. Let EAPs be armed with the knowledge of your services and the way they help the EAP.

Keep Your Name Familiar

Constantly look for opportunities to talk to gatekeepers about the value of your approach. The idea of presenting yourself repeatedly may be new to you. Because of a limited understanding of how marketing works, we have tended to believe that, once we told gatekeepers about our services or a new program, they would remember. If they then do not refer to us after this experiment in one trial learning, we tended to think that they must not like our ideas, or maybe they don't like us! NO! They just forgot.

Gatekeepers are busy. They are bombarded by demands for their attention all the time. It is easy for any of us to lose track of things. In addition, think about how this works with your therapy clients. When we are working with clients on significant change, we often go over the same ground repeatedly. The fact that many repetitions are needed is just the nature of change. Our marketing strategies need to respect this fact of life.

DEVELOPING A MARKETING PLAN

Now it is time to apply marketing concepts to your practice. Let's walk together through the process.

First, *select a service you want to offer*. Pick one that appeared on each of the first three lists in Chapter 7. This will mean that it is a service you know how to provide, it grabs your interest, and you have some reason to believe it speaks to a problem of urgent concern to some groups of people in your community. This belief will be based on the results of one of the three market studies we reviewed or on the basis of discussions with gatekeepers, or perhaps on a method you yourself developed to assess your market. Just be sure that your "market study" is not merely a projection of your wishes onto the community. Ideally the service you choose is one that will be easy for people to start. If you have a choice between marketing a 2-year psychoanalytic experience versus a 6-week marriage training course, pick the latter. If the 6-week program has value, some who take it will hang around for your 2-year program.

The service I plan to market is:

_____

_____

_____

Second, *identify your target group*. Who are the people who have the urgent concerns to which your service speaks? It is not everyone in the world. Identify who these people are. If you go with the marriage training course, the target group you think of first might be couples engaged to be married for the first time. If you keep thinking, you might come up with additional groups, such as:

- Divorced people who want to avoid repeating past mistakes
- Currently married people who want to strengthen their bond
- Maritally troubled people who want to avoid a divorce

Perhaps you will decide to target some combination of these groups. Now that you know who your target groups are, you do not have to worry about how to market to people who fall outside these categories. More importantly, a picture is building in your mind about who the people of interest are. As that picture becomes clearer, you will be able to figure out how to talk to them more effectively.

The target groups for my service are:

_____

_____

_____

_____

_____

Third, *articulate the value (benefits) your service will have for the target groups*. First-time marrieds have the value of wanting to stay happily married. They want to perpetuate the bliss and excitement of what they are currently experiencing. While that may not be possible in the literal sense, your training could help them to lay a stronger foundation for lifelong marriage by making the most of the bonding of the early years. That is a powerful value.

If your target groups include "the previously married," then the value may lie more in not repeating past mistakes. Most people want to have a significant other, and the sense of belonging, intimacy, affection, and normalcy that people perceive in a happy marriage. They want to avoid the intense emotional pain and financial disruption of another divorce. These are powerful values that your training may help to provide.

If your target groups include the maritally troubled, the value you offer could involve reestablishing the trust that existed before the marriage began to disintegrate. It could also involve avoiding the emotional pain and financial disruption of a divorce. These are also powerful values.

The potential values of my service to the target groups are:

_____

_____

_____

_____

_____

Fourth, *determine where you can find your target groups*. Suppose you want to target young engaged couples. Where do they hang out? The first thought may be a gatekeeper, such as the clergy who will perform the ceremony. We talked about joint programs with clergy as one possible service in Chapter 6. However, stretch your imagination. This is not the only narrow part of the funnel. Engaged couples also show up at bridal shops, tuxedo rental shops, hotels and other facilities that handle wedding receptions, department stores where they register for gifts, and so on.

What about divorced people? Where is their narrow part of the funnel? There are a number of support groups that cater to divorced people. Lawyers, judges, clergy, and family physicians come into contact with them regularly. They may read those "in search of" ads. Some may be in support groups for single parents. Perhaps there are magazines in your area that target singles as readers. Many decide to get back into shape and go to spas and athletic clubs. Some decide to drink their problems away, going to bars and clubs.

What about the currently married, whether troubled or not. Where is their narrow part of the funnel? Many couples attend church. One or both may be involved in the PTA or other school volunteer organizations. They get involved in youth groups, coaching children's sports, attending games and recitals. They take magazines such as *Parents Magazine*. They may be members of civic organizations.

The narrow part of the funnel for my targeted groups is:

_____

_____

_____

_____

_____

Fifth, *how can you best communicate with your target groups?* Historically, this is where most therapists have begun their marketing efforts. As you can see now, making such decisions without having done the previous spadework is likely to lead you to make ineffective choices. However, with the information you have now put together, you may already be getting ideas.

Much of this decision can be based on which narrow parts of the funnel you select. It makes little sense to use television ads for young engaged couples because they make up such a small percentage of the viewing audience. They make up a huge percentage of the clientele of bridal shops, however. Tasteful brochures or fliers that discuss your program that are provided through the bridal shop might be highly efficient. One challenge involves how to get the shop to cooperate. They might want to sell you their mailing list. Or they might see providing your information as a way of being of greater service to their clientele. Or you might be able to capture the imagination of the store owner as to the positive contribution your service provides to society. Look for an overlapping interest.

If you choose to go through the clergy, brochures and fliers are nice but the key is how your service may help solve a problem this gatekeeper has. One issue for clergy is keeping their congregation (read employers) happy. If your marriage training helps the clergy to be seen in a positive light by the congregation, then you are a long way toward home.

Suppose you decide to go after the divorced group. Speaking at their support groups (Suddenly Single, Parents Without Partners) is one idea. Always take material to leave with your audience. Such material should offer helpful hints and display your name, address, and phone number prominently. You could develop brochures or fliers that could be available at every meeting of the group. A tasteful ad near the "in search of" ads might also be effective.

What about married couples? Brochures and fliers distributed through the organizations they belong to and the professionals they consult are good. Speaking at these organizations can be useful. Two other strategies come to mind. One is to place an ad in local magazines that you have reason to believe may have many of these people as readers. In our area, the *Roanoker Magazine* is subscribed to by many of the same households that might get interested in learning more about marriage skills.

My wife came up with the following ad idea. Imagine a picture of two hands touching gently. New gold bands, candlelight, white flowers, tuxedo, and lace tell you that this is a special wedding picture. Beneath the picture are the words:

You were so happy then.
What went wrong?
What would you give to get it back?

In addition, my community has a company called Pin Point Marketing. If we have such a service in Roanoke, Virginia, I have to believe most urban centers do, as well. This company is a subsidiary of our newspaper. They deliver magazines and promotional material. They can help you select, with pinpoint precision, the neighborhoods you want to get your material. One approach is to "piggyback" with a magazine they deliver. Your flier or brochure can be delivered along with the magazine (perhaps *Parents Magazine,* or *Time,* or *Newsweek*) at 9 cents per piece. If you decide to select particular neighborhoods *en masse,* it will cost you 10 cents per piece.

Of course there is no law that says you can use only one method of communicating with potential clients. More, up to a point, is better. So you may do a combined set of strategies, such as arranging a variety of speaking engagements, connecting with a set of clergy to do team teaching, developing a brochure to be distributed by key stores and professionals, placing ads in carefully selected newspapers and magazines, and using your city's version of Pin Point Marketing.

The marketing tools that will be used in my campaign, and the reasons that they have been selected, are:

_____

_____

_____

_____

_____

As you develop your pieces of communication, what will you emphasize? Unless you skipped right to this page, you know that the answer is benefits. Describe benefits in language used by your target groups, not in words designed to impress your former graduate school professors. Keep the message honest and simple. Where possible, tell a story. Use graphics and pictures. Have a lot of "white space" — advertising code for "don't talk too much." Consult Levinson's (1993) *Guerrilla Marketing* for much of the technical information that will be useful to you in making your decisions.

Recently the American Psychological Association (APA) began a series of print ads designed to encourage people to use psychological services. These ads illustrate many of the points that have been made here. First and foremost, they speak to benefits. These benefits relate to matters of urgent concern to many readers, such as dealing with a troubled teenaged son, or responding to being downsized out of a job, or dealing with the emotional trauma of breast cancer. The ads' messages are conveyed in simple stories, using pictures of people with whom readers can identify. While the APA still endorses the concept that psychology is a health care profession, these ads do not raise that issue.

Sixth, *you must establish your credibility.* Executing the preceding five steps effectively will go a long way toward creating credibility. You will have established some credibility just by knowing where to reach people. You will have demonstrated your understanding of particular problems. How you run your office (review your business plan) will also help communicate your credibility. Look for tasteful ways to identify your training and experience that do not sound too "shrinky." In the wedding picture ad, for example, it could end with a simple listing of your name and title, degree, address and phone number.

The ways I will establish my credibility through my marketing tools are:

_____

_____

_____

During my "Building a Managed Care Free Practice" seminars, I walk participants through the development of a marketing plan around a particular service, just as you went through the six steps just now. At the end of the day, they break into groups. Each group comes up with a service and develops a marketing plan for it. The creativity that can be observed in this process gives me great faith in the future of our profession. Let me show you an example.

The service. One group came up with bereavement services for owners of pets that die. I must admit, as the group began its report, I thought they were reaching a bit far. By the time they finished, however, I could see it was brilliant. Since the first time, two other groups in other seminars have come up with the same service.

The market. In this case, it is easy to define potential users of the service — people whose pets have died or are in the process of dying. The fewer social supports they have, the more likely they are to need the service.

The value. People do get extremely attached to pets. Yet, although the feelings are real, people who grieve for a pet get far less social support than people who grieve for other losses. After a day or two, no one wants to hear about it, though in reality the feelings can last for some time. Some very lonely people have only pets for company. Their grieving may be overwhelming.

However, the problem, in and of itself, is circumscribed. Offering to help grieving pet owners is clearly less intrusive, and thus less threatening, than offering services around wholesale personality changes. It is an entry-level service that may very well lead to other reasons for consultation. Thus, it meets our criteria of relating to urgent concerns, having clear benefit, and being easy to start.

The narrow part of the funnel. Where do grieving pet owners congregate? Who has access to them? One clear answer is veterinarians. Most loving owners of sick pets have sought out veterinarian services. That is the easy answer. The group of seminar participants then came up with the harder answers: kennel clubs, dog and cat breeders, dog groomers, pet stores, pet boarders, pet trainers, pet sitting services, and pet cemeteries. Each of these is a potential access point to the target population.

Marketing methods to establish and communicate the value and your credibility. We could advertise in the newspaper because almost everyone takes the paper, and we are likely to reach grieving pet owners along with everyone else. However, newspaper ads can be expensive because of their broad distribution. Further, such ads lack a personal touch. Instead, imagine a flier (*repeatedly*) distributed at each of those points at the narrow part of the funnel. It could say something like:

The Loss of a Pet

Dr. Mary Stewart, psychologist, offers services to people who have lost a beloved pet. Too often, friends and family may not understand just how hard it is to lose a pet who has been part of our lives for many years. Maybe you live alone, and your pet was your main companion. Maybe you are a parent unsure how best to help your children with their first encounter with death. Maybe it just hurts. Dr. Stewart, herself an animal lover, helps adults and children deal with this difficult experience. Sometimes having a chance to talk with someone who knows how to help with these feelings can make a difference. Call 555-1234 to learn more or to make an appointment.

Mary Stewart, Ph.D.
123 Oak Lane
Suite 4
Roanoke, VA 24018

This flier establishes the value of the service. It gives readers a vision of what they might get from a consultation. It also establishes the therapist's credibility, both as a professional and as a human being. Value is further established by normalizing the experience rather than pathologizing it.

Sharing this flier with those likely to come into contact with grieving pet owners may win you some business. Why would such individuals want to help you? Because you are nice? Being nice will help but is insufficient. They will help you if it will help them solve their business problems. Veterinarians probably get little training in grief therapy and perhaps prefer to treat animals than listen to tears. They might appreciate having you take on a problem that they would rather not handle. Once a veterinarian believes in you, he or she may be willing to offer your flier to anyone who loses a pet. The veterinarian's endorsement will heighten your credibility. Those who operate kennel clubs, pet stores and cemeteries, as well as animal breeders, dog groomers, pet boarders, and so on, may also be willing to distribute or display your fliers because it helps them to serve their clientele better.

Once people have consulted you about their grief over their lost pets, they know you, and they will think of you when other difficult issues arise in their lives.

Measuring the results. Don't forget to measure the results of your marketing strategy. How many people show up to talk about losing pets? How did they hear about you? (Don't forget to ask.) After a year, you are likely to know which of the points on the narrow part of the funnel lead to referrals and which are not working out.

MARKETING STRATEGIES
FOR YOUR PRACTICE

Thus far we have been looking at methods of establishing a marketing strategy for a particular service. However, you may want to consider strategies that speak to your practice as a whole. These strategies can speak to particular services but also have the goal of familiarizing the community with your practice.

Yellow Pages

Look at your yellow pages ad in light of what we have been discussing. If you see what I saw in my own ad, and in therapists' ads I have examined all over the country, you will be disappointed. Most of our ads have focused on features, not benefits, and have employed language that creates barriers, either through jargon or by being (unintentionally) shaming.

For example, it is not uncommon to read ads of therapists who say they treat personality disorders. Who do you know that is willing to say: "Gee. I guess I do have a personality disorder. Maybe a couple of them"? However, I saw a yellow pages ad in Boise, Idaho, that I have shamelessly expropriated for myself. The ad offered services to people wanting to make "life pattern changes." Those words are a wonderful, shame-free reframe.

Most therapists' ads mention methods, focusing on their preferred types of therapy. Nobody cares. It is the goal (benefit) people are after. We need to let them see benefits in our ads.

I have changed my own yellow pages ad. My old ad committed the same mistakes as most therapists' ads. Let's compare:

Old Ad	New Ad
Ackley, Dana C. PhD–Licensed Clinical Psychologist– Psychotherapy for Children–Adolescents– Adults–Family–Marital– Group Therapy– Psychological Testing	**Ackley, Dana C. PhD–Licensed Clinical Psychologist–Problem solving/skill building for Children–Adolescents– Adults. Personal Performance Coaching– Life Pattern Changes**

My old ad emphasized methods or features. I can testify that it brought in few referrals. The only advantage my yellow pages ad has ever lent me is that, because my name begins with the letters "Ac" my listing is usually the first one in the category. Some of my colleagues have threatened to go into aardvark therapy. In my new ad, the titles still suggest services but in a way that potential clients can visualize benefits.

Over the years the yellow pages have not been a great source of referrals for therapists. Usually people learn about a therapist from a gatekeeper or by word of mouth. However, they may get several names and use the yellow pages to help them make a decision. In that way, the yellow pages may not introduce us to people, but they may help establish our credibility. In addition, as our market widens from its current 10% base toward the 100% goal, the yellow pages may become much more influential.

Speakers Bureau

Another step in acquainting the community with who you are is to maximize public-speaking opportunities. This is not a brand-new idea. Most of us have done our share of public speaking. However, some therapists are beginning to report that requests for talks are declining.

For those of you who want to utilize this technique, the answer is to be proactive. If you want speaking engagements, market yourself as a speaker. Use the same principles we have been discussing. Remember that the people looking for speakers have problems to solve. They must come up with someone to fill the speaking slot. Then they have to hope the person will have interesting things to say in an interesting way.

What can you do to fulfill these needs? First, work on your speaking style. We sometimes have the tendency to approach speaking engagements as if we were going to *lecture,* a speaking style best left in the college classroom. Your goal is to engage your audience, make them glad they came to hear you, and help them see you as someone with whom they could relate comfortably. You can make that happen by being pleasant, smiling, presenting material in easy to understand ways, making the material relevant to your audience, and having useful information for them to take home. Some additional advice:

- DO use audiovisuals, but make them interesting.
- DO NOT use overheads that look like a book page.
- DO NOT read your overheads to your audience—they can read. Rephrase your message or expand on your concepts.
- DO practice your presentation with someone willing to criticize it. What sounds wonderfully eloquent in our heads can sometimes bomb when it comes out of our mouths.

Second, consider the gatekeeper's problem of finding a presenter. Speak right to it. At the Manassas Group, we developed a brochure with the headline "Wondering Where You'll Find Your Next Speaker?" "We May Be Your Solution!" (See Figure 8.1.)

Third, you want your topics to reflect the overarching message that people can consult you about life's problems. They don't have to be "crazy" to see you. The topics our group developed for our brochure included:

- *No More Diets Please*
- *Living Well with Diabetes*
- *Mediation: An Alternative to Legal War*
- *Preventing Violence in Our Schools and Work Sites*
- *How to Help Children with Stress*
- *Helping Children Move from Pessimism to Optimism*
- *Conflict Management in the Workplace*
- *The Dollars and Sense of Psychology in Business*

FIGURE 8.1. Speakers Bureau brochure of the Manassas Group.

We had our brochure professionally designed by a graphic designer, which cost only a few hundred dollars more but resulted in an eye-catching design. Just as we want people to call on us for our professional expertise, we should consider using other professionals, when appropriate, as well.

Direct Mail

OK — maybe you want to call it "junk mail." But it is not really junk if it provides useful information about valuable services. People need to have ways that they can learn about what we have to offer. Direct mail offers an opportunity to provide that information. What gets passed off by some people as junk is another person's useful information. For example, how did you buy your last 10 professional books? My guess is that you learned about some, perhaps most, by direct mail.

Direct mail can be *directed* to your target groups. This selectivity increases the likelihood that recipients will see your material as valuable instead of junk. Suppose, for example, you decide to do a direct mailing about your service to grieving pet owners. One option to explore is whether kennel clubs sell their mailing lists. Pet food companies also may have mailing lists for sale.

What kinds of companies would sell their mailing lists? Is the practice ethical? Companies and organizations sell their mailing lists to increase revenues and provide their customers or members with additional useful information. The APA, state professional licensing boards, and *The Family Therapy Networker* are all examples of well-respected, highly ethical organizations that sell their mailing lists.

In addition, there are mailing list companies that specialize in putting together useful lists for marketers like you. They charge you a certain amount per name. You pay them for assembling the names and keeping a current list. They can sometimes arrange for your material to be sent by a company that prepares bulk mail. Such companies address the pieces and take them to the post office. However, you will still need to buy your own bulk-rate mail permit. You do this through your local post office. The permit costs about $85 per year, but you can save a fortune in postage. For example, when we mail out brochures for one of our seminars, it costs us just under 18 cents per piece rather than 32 cents. IMPORTANT TIP: Get instructions about how to prepare your material for mailing before you do it the first time. Bulk mail is a complicated process. Visit a customer service representative of the nearest business center of the Post Office. (Not all Post Offices have business centers.) That representative can provide you the necessary permits, forms, and publications. This step will save you considerable time, frustration, and expense.

As an alternative to bulk-rate mail, you might consider using companies like Pin Point Marketing that deliver material to target groups of interest to you. You could piggyback your materials with a relevant magazine, as discussed earlier. For example, if you are doing a piece to those grieving lost pets, you might piggyback with magazines directed toward pet owners, such as *Cat Fancy* and *Dog Fancy.*

Direct mail can be used to educate the community about your practice through newsletters, community canvases, and brochures. Each of these can be used to help the community develop a vision of using your services.

Newsletters

A newsletter can provide articles that focus on human problems, containing information that people would find helpful. If you write a useful piece on a problem of interest to readers, you have begun to establish your credibility as an expert in an area of potential urgent concern. Readers are likely to think: "This person understands my problem." This favorable impression can even spill over into other areas: "If he understands about subject A, maybe he can help with subject B." By writing about normal problems in living, you are helping to shift people's perceptions away from the image of a shrink who deals with mental illness to a more inviting, empowering image.

I believe strongly in the power of newsletters. The one I began in 1982 for referral sources doubtless saved my practice. It was designed to help referral sources solve problems with their own patients and clients. In the process, it helped them to see me as an expert in relevant areas. Beyond that, it reminded them that I existed. They too are bombarded by 2,700 marketing messages a day.

Some people say that newsletters don't work. It is true that some newsletters do not work. It is my personal opinion that a well-written, locally produced newsletter that is closely crafted for a carefully targeted audience can do a lot of good. I have less faith in mass-produced newsletters that are sold to therapists to be distributed to the public. My objection to them is that they cannot have the personal touch. They provide readers with much less of an experience of being with the therapist who distributes them. Again, this is an opinion of mine, and you may feel differently.

Let's suppose that you or your practice group decides that the idea of a newsletter is attractive. However, you may feel that it is too expensive. You, your group, and other therapists in your community could form a marketing guild to publish a newsletter. Ivan Miller, Ph.D., a psychologist in Boulder, Colorado, has founded such a guild and offers guidance about how guilds like these can be established (see the Appendix for his address and phone number).

Your newsletter could come out quarterly, distributed by an outfit like Pin Point Marketing as well as through the offices of gatekeepers with which you have good relationships. Its goal would be to help the community identify you as someone who provides Problem-Solving/Skill-Building services. Your newsletter could have issues on such topics as teaching children about work, building family self-esteem, gender differences, and the hurried/harried family. Let's consider the rationale behind these particular topics.

The first one, teaching children about work, lets parents know that you have information and skills useful to them in raising children. In this case, we are talking about helping children to learn that work exists in the world. Certainly, all parents must teach their children about work. Since most people were raised on the nagging method, that is what most parents use in their work-educative efforts. Yet, no parent is really satisfied with this approach. A newsletter issue devoted to this topic could offer some alternatives, establishing your credibility in this area.

Second, consider family self-esteem. It is hard to go wrong with self-esteem. By orienting the issue toward families instead of just children, you can involve a wider audience. This approach moves you away from just parenting issues and introduces "something for everyone." In this way, the newsletter can help the therapists in your group or guild who work with children while simultaneously establishing the credibility of the adult therapists, as well.

Thanks to John Gray (*Men Are from Mars, Women Are from Venus*), we know that people are highly interested in learning about gender issues today. In this case, we do not even have to visit the bookstore. We can just read the best-seller list and listen to what our clients talk about. A newsletter can show that you are a resource in sorting out gender-based conflicts.

Finally, almost every family I see tells me about their overly crowded schedules. Two careers, baseball games, PTA meetings, karate classes, and a wealth of other activities define the typically frenetic pace of living in an opportunity-rich society. Too many people see themselves as failures unless they take advantage of all the opportunities. They need a way out from under this false burden of guilt. A newsletter issue devoted to this topic can let them know that you can help them to find it.

In addition to a main article, a newsletter could have some other features. Ideally, a newsletter will invite the reader to take action. Therefore, in the interest of making it easy for readers to initiate a relationship, consider giving a free 30-minute consultation to readers who complete a four-question quiz on the newsletter's topic. Second, in the interest of creating credibility and greater name familiarity, be sure to list the names of all therapists who are sharing the cost of the newsletter. Finally, brief descriptions of special or new services that members provide can be included. Box 8.3 shows a newsletter prototype.

BOX 8.3. Newsletter for a Therapist Group:
Prototype Article

THE CONSULTANT

A publication of the Family Consultation Center

The Consultant *is written to provide information to the community about handling problems in our stressful times. Its writers are members of the Family Consultation Center, an association of licensed professionals who work with people on personal, family, and work issues.*

TEACHING CHILDREN ABOUT WORK

It is a crystal clear, mild November Saturday. Neighbors Fred Gardner and Don Blackwell are enthused about getting out in the fresh air to get their leaves raked. In the process, both will involve their children. Only Blackwell is going to have a nice day.

As Gardner leaves the breakfast table, his 6-year-old daughter asks to "help," calling her 7-year-old brother as well. Fred sighs but gamely allows the children to join him. At first, things are not too bad as the three are caught up in the beautiful weather. But soon the neighborhood reverberates with Fred's reprimands. The children had been playing in the leaves. When the shouting starts, so does the complaining. "We hate raking leaves!" both children scream. Fred is determined to make them finish the task, to teach them about work. The kids eventually win by doing the job so poorly that he finally sends them to their rooms, crying.

Blackwell is greeted with a similar request from his children. He grins, does a rapid recalculation of how his morning will go, and agrees to have their "help." The Blackwell yard also reverberates with noise, but it is the noise of happy squeals and Don's shouted excitement over his children's efforts. What does Don know that Fred does not?

All parents have to teach their children about work. Every parent dreads it. "It's easier to do it myself!" is a parental mantra. While teaching children about work is not easy, there are three steps parents can take to give themselves a fighting chance.

1. **Remember this is a two-part task:** Don's "rapid recalculation" was to realize that he now had two jobs, not just one. This morning,

(cont.)

(*continued from previous page*)

he was not just going to get leaves raked. Now he was going to rake leaves *and* teach his children about work. By shifting his expectations, he minimized the disappointment he would feel when the leaf job was not done with adult efficiency and neatness. He could allocate energy to both tasks. Much of Fred's frustration was based on inaccurate expectations. It is natural to get frustrated when things don't go as we plan.

Children are not born with the Work Ethic. We must create opportunities to teach it to our children. When we remember that this is part of our role, we will plan to devote enough of our energy toward it.

2. **Have age-appropriate expectations of what children can do:** Fred was confused about what his children could do. Like many parents, he tended to view small children as totally helpless. Then, after a certain age, he believed that they should have an adult's ability to know what constitutes a "good job."

Fred did not quite realize these were his thoughts because they were assumptions, ideas that get developed early in life, when we have not yet fully matured. We sometimes forget to question them when we get older. All of us make assumptions, and some of them are accurate. However, we only know the degree of their accuracy if we question them sometimes.

Fred's assumptions were unfortunate. Young children are not helpless. In fact, they are thrilled to be learning new skills and eager to show off to their parents. Reasonable chores can help to build skills and a feeling of pride of accomplishment. Overwhelming chores create a sense of failure.

Don more accurately estimated his children's abilities. For example, he knew that, at their age, their ability to sustain energy for this job might be an hour or so. He knew he would be finishing alone. When they began to complain of "being tired," he pushed the limits but only a little. He said: "You two have done a great job so far. I want you to finish that one area over there and that will be enough." He heard some groans, but the kids and he both knew the additional work was manageable, not overwhelming.

3. **Remember that children don't think like adults:** Children get confused by many things adults find easy to understand. This is because they have not had enough life experience to be able to think in the abstract terms that adults take for granted. "I love you," an abstract statement adults understand, is pretty meaningless for children without hugs, kisses, praise, protection, feeding, and discipline.

(*cont.*)

(continued from previous page)

"Rake the leaves neatly," likewise, doesn't mean much to young children. One child may nod earnestly and then hold the rake primly; another will rake so he doesn't get any spots on his clothes; a third may panic because leaves keep getting stuck to her rake, making it look messy. Still others will think neatness means whatever they are corrected for most often: A noisy boy may rake quietly, and a slowpoke will rake quickly.

Fred, seeing the children's nods, assumed his children knew what the abstract term "neat" meant and interpreted their subsequent behavior as willful disobedience. This fed his anger, which fed his children's belief in their incompetence.

Don knew that he had to tie "neat" to actual experience. He had to offer concrete training in what he meant. He did so in two ways. First, he demonstrated neatness in his own raking. In the long run doing what you want your children to do is the most powerful parental teaching technique. Second, he caught his children being neat. It wasn't easy. Initially, he had to settle for the beginnings of an approximation of neatness. When he saw it, he said: "Wow! You are starting to do some really neat leaf raking!" Then he added: "Uh-Oh. I see some stragglers over there. Let's go get them." And together they did.

In all honesty, not all of Don's work lessons went so smoothly. He had moments of frustration and despair too. They are inherent in the process of teaching children about work. However, on balance, by using the three ideas discussed here, he helped his children grow up to be more competent and have a greater sense of pride and accomplishment.

It is easy for parents to get stuck in an unproductive cycle trying to teach our children about work. It comes up with household chores and in the dreaded area of homework. The professionals who staff the Family Consultation Center have many years of experience helping parents and children get "unstuck." Please feel free to call if we can be of service.

Notice that the article is written in normal language. It is not about the Family Consultation Center. It is about the parents who will read the article. Parents have no interest whatsoever in reading about the Family Consultation Center. They want to read about themselves, which this article is designed to let them do. If they experience any benefit whatsoever in reading this newsletter, the credibility of The Family Consultation Center increases, as does the chance of their getting a call from frustrated parents.

Community Canvas

Another direct mail possibility is a community canvas. It offers a one-step method to accomplish the two steps of marketing. It asks the community for information so that you can get educated about your potential clients' interests. However, the questions themselves convey information (much like the speaking topics in the Manassas Group's brochure for the Speaker's Bureau). The questions in the canvas (see Box 8.4 for a prototype) provide the community with a new way to view your services. The idea of the community canvas is to get people to try you out. Once they have had a chance to establish a relationship with you, who knows what directions your work together may take.

The specific topics you might list in a canvas would vary, depending on your clinical interests and the interests of others in your group. The list in this canvas is long enough to represent many of the diverse interests of our profession. It may be too long. It is presented to you as an untested prototype that requires further development. The hope is that it will generate some experiments.

The explanation of the service formats gives people a description of what they may experience, presented in non–mental illness terms. Many people are put off by the word "therapy" — and to them an even worse word is "psychotherapy." This development is distressing to many of us because we have an emotional attachment to the name of an activity we see as high status (for us). Regular people do not seem to like it. The formats give people some choices about how to work with us in ways they find most comfortable.

Brochures for Specific Services

In addition to newsletters and canvasses, which are more general types of marketing, you can use direct mail to market a specific service. Suppose you wanted to market a service to graduating high school seniors and their parents. This transition is a time of anxiety and missteps for many families. You could buy a mailing list of graduating seniors in your area and mail a brochure outlining your service.

Your Marketing Budget

Marketing will require that you spend money. Some expenses will be direct expenses, such as getting material printed and distributed, paying for ads

BOX 8.4. Community Canvas Prototype

Dear Member of the Roanoke Valley:

The XYZ Group would like to expand the services we offer to the community, and we would like your help in designing them.

Until recently, our services focused on problems covered by insurance because most people used insurance to pay our fees. We have come to realize that this is a mistake because using insurance in this way creates problems. It allows insurance companies, instead of you, the consumer, to decide what services are provided. Artificial limits are set about who can use our services and how long people can see us. These problems have gotten worse with the advent of managed care.

One problem that worries us about using insurance benefits today is the serious compromise made with regard to privacy. Employers, insurance companies, and managed care companies all justify learning about visits because they have some role in authorizing the money for payments. The 700 insurance companies that belong to the Medical Information Bureau pool information they gather among all their members.

We still **can** *offer privacy to people who decide to pay for services themselves rather than using insurance. Under those circumstances, no reports are made to anyone. People can talk to us for as long as they wish by themselves, as a couple or as a family. People do not have to have a psychiatric diagnosis. The kinds of problems we can discuss do not have to fit some insurance company's ideas of what our services are for.*

This means that our services can be much more flexible and creative. They can be much more about the real-life issues that bring most people into our offices. In our fast-paced, high-demand society, everyone is constantly faced with new challenges. No one has all the life experiences needed to meet every possible challenge. We specialize in helping people solve new problems and build new skills.

The best services we can offer to you are the ones that fit the problems you face. By answering the attached questionnaire, you can help us design our new services to fit the real needs of our community. Of course, we ask you to respond anonymously. If you want more information, please feel free to call our offices to talk with one of us.

(cont.)

(continued from previous page)

QUESTIONNAIRE

Please circle the items that are relevant to you and/or your family.

Family issues:

1. Overly stressed children
2. Overly stressed adolescents
3. Overly stressed adults
4. Overly hurried family: too much to do, too little time.
5. Jobs interfere with family living
6. Too much sibling rivalry
7. Underachievement in school
8. Problems making children mind
9. Children adjusting to divorce
10. Making stepparent relationships work

Adult issues:

11. Making marriage work
12. Improving an OK marriage
13. Finding a spouse
14. Adjusting to being single again

15. How to be a visited parent
16. Reestablishing the family meal
17. Weight control
18. Learning to handle conflict
19. Developing psychological resiliency
20. Dealing with aging parents

Work issues:

21. Finding the right career
22. Handling a difficult boss
23. Learning to say "no" to the job
24. Handling sexual harassment on the job
25. Performing well under pressure
26. Changing the work culture
27. Two-career families
28. Setting priorities
29. Underachieving on the job

We plan to offer services in three formats: *exclusive, interactive, and classroom-style.* Descriptions of each format follow. Please consider these formats in light of the circled topics that interest you most.

I. The Exclusive Format

This format is private and individually tailored to fit your situation: individuals, couples, families, or work groups. Only you or the people of your choice who are directly involved in your situation are present. You discuss all your issues in strict confidentiality.

(cont.)

(*continued from previous page*)

Factors to consider

- Time and effort of the consultations are entirely concentrated on your issues.
- Absolute privacy is guaranteed. This is reassuring should there be any highly personal issues you would like to discuss. No one, including insurance companies and your employer, will know your business.
- Most expensive format.
- Other formats provide more potential sources of input.

II. The Interactive Small-Group Format

This format offers hands-on, small-group discussion and exercises designed to speak to relevant issues of the group. You can sign up by topic. Your group will include people with the same interests or concerns as you have. This format offers the opportunity to discuss topics of concern, seek out new methods to handle old problems, and exchange ideas with others concerned about the same issue(s). This method uses the power of group interaction to generate real answers. Meet people with similar concerns, or form your own group—get a group of people together and request sessions on a topic of your choice. For example, a group of parents concerned about teenage dating or teenage drinking (or both) might request a brief series of meetings.

Factors to consider

- Less expensive than the **Exclusive Format.**
- Lots of input from people in similar situations.
- "Guided synergy"—a combination of energy and ideas from people highly invested in the topic and in finding solutions to tough problems. Bounce ideas off each other. The group is kept productive and goal-directed by a skilled moderator with advanced training in behavioral science.
- May not be as well suited to some personal, private material, though it can be if the group agrees.
- While some may perceive having to share time as a disadvantage, the richness of the interactions often provides experiences not available in the **Exclusive Format.**

(*cont.*)

(*continued from previous page*)

III. Classroom-Style Seminars

These are classes lasting 4–12 weeks, depending on the topic. They are more content focused and less interactive. There is less opportunity to work on individual concerns in class. You use the information learned in class to work on issues at home or on the job.

Factors to consider

- Least expensive format.
- Lots of formal, organized, in-depth material presented on your topic by an experienced professional in the behavioral sciences.
- Least interactive format, which some may prefer.
- Least chance to address individual issues in class (i.e., participants would not ordinarily focus on their individual situations and individual solutions).

Please tell us which formats seem best for your circled issues. List the number of each topic you circled beside the format you would prefer to use with it.

Exclusive: _____

Interactive: _____

Classroom: _____

Would our new way of offering services make it more likely that you would come to see us? If not, what could we add or change?

_____

_____

_____

_____

Thank you for your help.

in newspapers or magazines, buying mailing lists, getting layout and logo design services, and so forth. Other expenses will involve your time. Like your money, your time is a limited resource. How can you best use it? Writing brochures, giving talks, and meeting with gatekeepers are all potentially useful.

In deciding how to spend your limited time and money, think like a business person. Do not focus on cost. Focus on value. What value can you get for your investment? Notice that this is the same question your potential clients will be asking about your services. Levinson and Godin, in their book *The Guerrilla Marketing Handbook* (1994), a companion piece to *Guerrilla Marketing* (Levinson, 1993), tell the story of a Manhattan therapist trying to establish her practice. The marketing project she conducted led to $7,200 in fees over the course of a year. This was based on mailing 500 letters to a well-defined group with a relevant service. It led to 40 phone calls, 25 participants in a get-acquainted session, and 3 people who eventually came for sessions.

Some might be discouraged that only three people became clients. They are looking at the wrong results. The financial return was well in excess of the time and money spent. In addition, the word-of-mouth payoff of those 22 people who did not happen to choose to come for services *right now* could prove tremendous in the long run.

SUMMARY

This chapter is not intended to be the last word on marketing. It is intended to get you started by showing you the basics and helping you to figure out how to use them in an ethical, practical, and effective manner. From here you can consult such resources as Levinson's *Guerrilla Marketing* to take you to the next level.

Summary for Part II

The task for Part I was to fire your imagination and your energy. The task of Part II was to give you specific ways to use your energy to implement the new model and ideas. As you do so, remember the following:

- The three building blocks of a successful business (practice) are knowing what people want or need, letting them know you have it, and making it easy for them to start their relationship with you.
- Using the Problem-Solving/Skill Building model can open your mind to a sea of opportunities and new ways you can serve your communities.
- A carefully constructed business plan will guide you through the unavoidable times of confusion and anxiety. Following the form in Chapter 7 will lead you to answer the key questions.
- Marketing involves educating yourself about the community and the community about you. Marketing can be done well within the ethical boundaries of our profession.

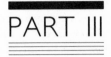

PART III

DIVERSIFYING YOUR SERVICES: TAKING YOUR SKILLS TO THE WORKPLACE

Several years ago, the orange juice people tried a new approach to their marketing. They wanted to broaden people's perception of how to use their product, so in their ads they told us, "Orange juice. It's not just for breakfast anymore." We need to find ways to make a similar point: Personal learning about problem solving and skill building is not just for people with DSM diagnoses anymore.

The goal of this book is to give you ways to sell your skills outside the arena of third-party payment. Thus far, we have examined ways to develop and market our traditional services. Now it is time to consider other ways people can use our expertise. Diversification is important to us because it increases the chances that we can generate enough income to sustain our practices without third parties and their controls. It is important to those who use our services because a broader range of useful services will be available to them.

When I decided to forgo managed care opportunities, I did a lot of research. I thought long and hard about how to do private pay therapy. The plans that I developed made sense to me. Still, there were many unknowns. The one fact I knew was that I was unwilling to leave my future to chance. The more applications of my skills that I could use in my practice, the greater safety my practice would have. Therefore, I looked for additional ways to use those skills that would help me to maintain my independence.

I found that many of my skills could be applied to work settings for the benefit of both employees and employers. I call this expansion of service "People-Consulting in the Workplace." It fits the criteria needed for a managed care free practice because: (1) it is paid for directly, not through a third party; (2) it speaks to urgent needs most people have; (3) it provides a large segment of our population direct access to our expertise; (4) it serves to *normalize* our services; and (5) it offers strong financial rewards. As my experience grows, I am finding it an exciting and rewarding diversification. That is why I have developed it here for you in detail.

Of course, People-Consulting in the Workplace is not the only diversification open to you. Diversifications exist *wherever* people have human problems to solve and skills to build. Behavioral medicine is one example of a diversification that offers high value to its users. Further, eliminating the issue of mental illness from our services when we work with behavioral and emotional factors of physical healing is a powerful contribution to well-being. There are hundreds of potential services in behavioral medicine alone. Forensics and sports psychology are other diversifications that come to mind.

Regardless of the choices you make about diversification, as you increasingly take the Problem-Solving/Skill-Building perspective, you will find that the field is much more seamless than it has appeared. You are an agent of human change. There are applications of those skills to be found wherever humans operate. There will be specific content-based skills and knowledge to acquire, but shifting your self-definition from mental illness treater to being an agent of human change creates a world of opportunities.

To illustrate, when I am doing therapy, by using the skills developed by my training and experience, I am an agent of human change. When I provide consultation to business through People-Consulting in the Workplace, I am an agent of human change. Finally, when I do my own seminars or provide consultations to therapists about their practices, I am an agent of human change. In each of these three situations, my goal is to help people (therapy clients, employers/employees, seminar participants) to solve problems of urgent concern and to build their skills.

Chapter 9 explains People-Consulting in the Workplace and then deals with many of the issues we need to think through in developing this area. Chapter 10 identifies some of the services that fall within the broad range of our skills. Its goal is to stimulate your imagination. Chapter 11 helps you develop a business plan for this diversification. Finally, Chapter 12 introduces the processes of marketing and selling these services.

Chapter 9

New Applications for Your Skills: People-Consulting in the Workplace

People-Consulting in the Workplace is the application of the Problem-Solving/Skill-Building model to the human issues in the workplace that keep people from feeling and doing their best on the job. Such issues include how people get along with one another, how power is handled, how people communicate with each other, how people deal with the natural and sometimes excessive stress of jobs, how people respond to traumas that sometimes happen at work, and a myriad of other human issues about which we are experts.

People-Consulting in the Workplace recognizes that employees are people, and that, as such, they each bring their own psychological strengths and weakness to work. It recognizes that company leaders also bring their personal limitations to the extremely challenging task of getting a diverse group of people pulling in the same direction. It deals with the interaction of intrapersonal, interpersonal, and systemic issues. Everyone, at all levels of a company, is a candidate for our services. Overcoming barriers to optimal work performance is a never ending task, just as is overcoming the barriers to personal growth.

Lou Perrott and I offer our People-Consulting in the Workplace services through our consultation firm, Peak Performance Consultation. Its mission statement is: "We deal with the psychological barriers to productivity." This statement identifies our focus. It establishes our value to our clients by speaking to an area of urgent concern, productivity. Employee productivity is the *key* to profit in business, which of course is the fundamental urgent concern. Raising employee productivity even a small amount can do great things for a company's profitability. The mission statement also shows our flexible approach. Rather than touting a method, we work to solve the problem, using whatever method or resources are appropriate to the situation.

Our mission statement leaves us available to handle psychological barriers to productivity that may have a variety of sources. For example, a company may have a department that is experiencing operating difficulties, which might arise from such causes as:

- A leader whose leadership or interpersonal skills are underdeveloped
- A hidden conflict that needs airing
- A rebellious culture that has evolved within the department
- External forces preventing the department from getting the resources it needs
- A member having suffered a terrible on-the-job accident, leaving a set of traumatized coworkers
- A company-wide morale problem
- Inadequate training

And there are other possibilities. Our task is to listen and respond to the problem rather than to rely on a set of canned responses. Our job is to figure out what is going on and then help to develop and implement a solution. Sometimes we train. Sometimes we troubleshoot. Sometimes we coach individuals. Sometimes we help people reestablish trust and communication. Sometimes we help them find additional problem-solving resources.

WHAT PEOPLE-CONSULTING IN THE WORKPLACE IS NOT

- People-Consulting in the Workplace is not EAP work. We are not talking about finding deeply troubled people on the job so that we can provide screening and treatment. That would be pursuing the 10% market. We are after the 100% market.
- It is not simply doing traditional psychotherapy at a different site. While People-Consulting in the Workplace makes use of our skills and training, it differs from what we usually do, one on one, in our offices. Some adaptations are necessary and will be discussed later.

- People-Consulting in the Workplace is not the highly technical work of industrial psychologists, such as job analysis, performance appraisal systems, compensation programs, or ergonomics (the psychological aspects of engineering). There are many aspects of industrial psychology that are far different from anything within our realm of knowledge.
- Finally, People-Consulting in the Workplace is not just organizational development. While there are some areas of overlap, there are also activities that belong uniquely within the organizational development realm and some that are uniquely based in People-Consulting.

Some of you may be tempted to think already that People-Consulting in the Workplace is not for you. When we do our seminars, there are always several participants who assume that this particular diversification is not for them. Perhaps they cannot imagine their interests overlapping with this area, they feel intimidated, or they choose to exclude themselves from the business world because of an ingrained belief that business equals exploitation of workers. Most (though not all) of these participants change their minds as we go through the material.

I invite you to do what they do: Keep an open mind as you read about People-Consulting in the Workplace, and then decide. Write down your concerns and fears now (see Box 9.1). Some questions that seminar participants typically raise have included: Can the values of business be consistent with our values? Do we really have the skills? How do I get started? How do I get into a company? What should I charge? If the company pays me, how do I earn employee trust? Do I need more training? If so, what? If the company pays me to work with employees, isn't that a form of third-party payment? Usually we cover these questions to everyone's satisfaction. Let's see how well the rest of our discussion about People-Consulting in the Workplace does in speaking to *your* issues.

ETHICAL ISSUES IN WORKING WITH BUSINESS, OR . . . WHAT'S A NICE GIRL LIKE YOU DOING IN A PLACE LIKE THIS?

Let's begin with the question of values. Can our values and business values coexist, even come to cooperate? Many people, not just therapists, see business as based on cutthroat competition, a game in which there are winners and losers. This mentality *sometimes can be seen* in how businesses compete with one another and in how management treats its employees. However, it probably has never been as widespread as some of us have believed. Just as business people often misread our culture, we

---

**BOX 9.1. My Questions and Concerns about Doing
"People-Consulting in the Workplace"**

_____

_____

_____

_____

_____

_____

_____

_____

_____

_____

---

are vulnerable to misreading theirs. More importantly, the business culture has been changing, for highly practical reasons. It is more profitable to think more humanely these days.

Business today is engaging in much more "win–win" thinking. Thus, as business deals are made, and as employers and employees figure out how to relate to each other, the most successful businesses are learning that both parties need to leave the table with something positive. If one party loses, it will be hard to do business again in the future. If both parties profit, they know and trust each other. It will be easier to do business in the future.

> A couple came to my office to work on their marriage. The man was a highly successful salesman. The couple engaged in the typical competitive, controlling types of behavior that drive so many couples apart. They were focused on win–lose. One day I asked the salesman, "Who wins when you sell something to a client?" "We both do!" he replied without hesitation. Repeat business and maintaining relationships are crucial to his success. That meant that his clients need to get something of value for their money while the salesman has to earn a fair commission. When I suggested he could apply that same mentality to his marriage, it was like a light went on in his head.

Such thinking is on the rise in business. Employers are learning that, when the interests of both employers _and employees_ are kept strongly in mind, operations run more smoothly. There is voluminous data to support this conclusion. Bob Rosen is one of the pioneers in this form of psychological consultation in the workplace. He was trained as a clinical psychologist but has been consulting to business and industry for the past decade. He began his career as a therapist for adolescents, often working with the children of Type-A executives. He began to wonder: "If these people are creating such havoc with their families, what are they doing to people at work?" Finding the answer to that question led him into full-time consulting to business.

One of the fruits of his work is his book *The Healthy Company* (1991). In it, he presents extensive evidence of how employee and employer well-being overlap. Traditionally, the relationship between management and workers has been adversarial, based on the false notion that they were engaged in a zero-sum game in which there were only $X to be had. Every dollar that goes to employees is thought to be lost to management. The truth is that, when companies attend constructively to human issues, $X becomes $X +. Rosen's book demonstrates that the most profitable companies in America are those that pay effective attention to people issues in the workplace.

Supporting Rosen's work are the results of a business study reported by the Associated Press (1995) conducted by the management consulting firm Ernst & Young LLP for the U.S. Department of Labor. They found that companies that treat employees as assets, and invest in training and other employee benefit programs, are more profitable than other companies. Within that study, for example, Motorola Inc. estimated it earns $30 for every $1 invested in training. Xerox Corp. said that cooperation between management and unions had reduced manufacturing costs by 30% and had cut the time needed to develop new products by half.

Upon reflection, these findings make sense. Companies are going to do best when working conditions are designed to support higher-level psychological functioning, which can only surface in an atmosphere of win–win. Cutthroat competition brings out the worst in people. Building something together in a manner in which both parties can do well brings out the best. It is synergistic.

This does not mean that it is easy to make cooperation happen. Executives (many of whom may lack the extensive knowledge of human issues that we bring to the table) may not know what many of these desirable conditions are. For example, they often do not know that fear is a powerful motivator *only in the short term*. They may not recognize that conflict avoidance only hides issues, making them more difficult to manage in the long run, or more prone to blow up unexpectedly in the future. No one may have told them that trauma in the workplace often creates terrible barriers to productivity. Few of us have been there to help company leaders learn about these and other issues.

Some of you may worry about the potential corruption of our own values with regard to the conflict between helping and materialism. Can we keep our virtue in the land of greed? Will we slowly sell out our principles to chase the almighty dollar? If we do, we might as well stay with managed care. One simply cannot make enough money to fill the void left by abandoning one's conscience. However, sometimes we have thought we were responding to conscience when in reality we were responding to prejudice and self-doubt. We will have a much better chance of holding onto an appropriate value system if we separate fact from fiction.

A common perception among us has been that we are working for the good of society while business seems to be working just for itself. This view might actually be more polemical than accurate. It feeds the worry that, if we allow ourselves to become involved in business issues, we will lose our ability to advance social good.

In reality, all people, not just us, have to struggle with the issue of balancing self-interests and working to better our society. We looked at our struggles with this issue in Chapter 3. Everyone has responsibilities to society, and we all have responsibilities to attend to our own self-interests. People sometimes make the mistake of overemphasizing one or the other set of responsibilities. When *we* make mistakes, we are more likely to ignore our own self-interests. This tendency puts us in danger of developing a most unattractive identity, that of the long-suffering martyr.

We perceive business people as too often making the mistake of overemphasizing self-interest. Some do. But most business people make some attempt to create a balance, just as most people everywhere do. Businesses in my community often make substantial donations to charity. Many of them "loan" executives to the United Way. It is in the culture of many businesses to encourage their leaders to get involved in the community. In fact, it seems to me that this is much more frequent behavior among people involved in business than it is among therapists.

However, overt good works aside, business contributes to the social good by its very existence. The computer I am typing on was made by a business. Because that business decided to go to the trouble, expense, and *risk* of making this product, it became available for me to purchase. I am now free to use it to advance my own interests. In the meantime, that company took the money I paid for my computer and used it. It paid employees so that they could support themselves and their families. It bought parts from other companies, allowing the employees of those companies to make a living. The owners of this computer company probably make a sizable income, perhaps inspiring others to start businesses that will, in turn, create new products that the public might want or need. All of these things advance the public good. One role of business is to provide us with things that we want, enjoy, learn from, and/or need.

Another role of business is to create wealth. "Wealth" is a word that makes many of us uncomfortable. In this case, I do not mean making a few people gazillionaires, although this is one side effect of the free market system. In this context, I am using wealth to refer to the economic well-being of the broad middle class. This wealth is fundamental to providing people with relative safety, education, diverse opportunities for achievement, and the context within which increasing numbers of people can have the chance to approach self-actualization.

Can businesses be abusive and unethical? Of course. We know that some businesses and business people get so caught up in making a profit that they forget other values in the equation. We now know that this actually costs them profits. Can therapy be misused and conducted in an unethical manner? We know the answer to that all too well. But, we would not want our reputations to be determined by the bad actors in our profession—any more than we should base all of our perceptions of the business community on their bad actors.

Further, consider this. Do we require that our therapy clients always behave appropriately before we will agree to work with them? Of course not. If a sociopathic person wanted therapy to help him be a better con man, most of us would decline the offer. However, if someone who had acted badly wanted our help in changing his pattern of behavior, it would be easy to say yes. We do so all the time.

Finally, it may help us to get past our biases if we think about the many therapy clients we have who are business people. These are real people, and we can see in them the full range of their humanity. It is easy for us to lose this range of vision when we lump people together into categories.

In the long run, we will find that the business and therapy communities have much to teach each other. Perhaps we will add to our knowledge of appropriate self-interest from better understanding the value system of business. Perhaps business will learn about human issues from us. Each community will be the better for it, and each will profit.

BUT WHAT ABOUT . . . ?

Before we leave this discussion, let's look at some specific issues that may trouble you as you consider entering the world of business and profit.

Downsizing

Business decisions sometimes seem to hurt people. Downsizing, for example, is a particularly troublesome event. When we read about companies laying off large numbers of employees, it is easy to imagine that the company does not care about its people. Indeed, some companies behave in ways that seem to validate that impression.

Thus, the idea of actually helping a company do downsizing, which will get discussed, may seem to be an immoral act. Perhaps our role should be to talk leaders out of downsizing, thereby helping employees to avoid the emotional disruption and pain that any downsizing will cause. Sometimes, this may be a valid approach. Perhaps through process consultation we could help the company's leaders discover alternative ways to solve the company's problems.

However, businesses go through cycles of life and death, growth and cutback, just as people do. Sometimes downsizings really must be done. We know from our clinical experience that we cannot always prevent bad things from happening. Marriages end. Parents abuse. Exams are failed. We can, however, help people to cope with bad events more successfully than they would have without our help. In the case of downsizings, we can help executives who really must reduce the size of their companies to do so in humane ways.

Let's look at it from the leader's perspective for a moment. As an employer myself, I have had to fire two people for cause. Each time was terribly unpleasant. I can only imagine how much more painful it is to take someone's job who has been performing well. Figuring out how to handle your feelings in that situation must be a difficult human problem. Most people have not had the opportunity to develop their skills in solving that problem. Maybe we could help them do so. After all, we have helped countless people identify and handle their feelings in many other difficult human situations. As you will see, the more company leaders are in touch with and express their feelings in this situation, the more humanely downsizings can be accomplished.

We could also work with companies to develop programs that help survivors to deal with the difficult feelings inherent even in humanely effected reductions in workforce. Finally, if we make ourselves available, we can help casualties of downsizing to work through their understandable grief in the most efficient way possible so that they can get back on their work feet.

We cannot offer these services while maintaining the naive attitude that downsizing is always wrong. It may always be sad, but it is not always wrong. A company that really must reduce its size will go out of business if it does not recognize and act on that need. What happens to the employees who would have survived a downsizing *then*? We cannot be emotionally available to help company leaders with these difficult situations if we keep ourselves in a position of moral smugness.

Individual Employee Dismissal

In addition to downsizings, businesses also occasionally dismiss or fire individual employees. This is an emotionally laden event for all concerned. Because many people in supervisory positions do not have good access to their feelings, such situations often get mishandled. Often, the problems that trigger dismissals are initially ignored. Irritations grow. Ineffective discussions are held in which communication is inadequate. Finally, the supervisor fires the person after "one screwup too many." Legal problems often ensue for the company. What could have been handled on an emotional level gets handled at the legal level. Worse yet, we read increasingly about workplace violence perpetrated by people who have been fired. Might not some of tomorrow's legal imbroglios or workplace violence be prevented through improved interpersonal skills for supervisors?

Suppose you were working with a supervisor to help her develop her ability to communicate. Suppose you were training her to recognize how her feelings of frustration were mixed with anxiety over her underdeveloped skills in influencing behavior. Suppose you helped her to develop assertiveness skills, which she could then use to work with the inadequately performing employee. A direct or indirect consequence might be that the employee's job could be salvaged.

Sometimes, a job cannot be salvaged. Sometimes a person is just in the wrong job, one that does not suit his or her talents. When this kind of hiring mistake is made, it can be handled in one of two ways. The more common way is for the supervisor, out of anxiety, to communicate to the employee that he is a loser: "You're just not getting the job done. I can't let this go on. I tried to warn you, but you've left me no choice!" (The supervisor's private, internal dialogue may be something more like "It makes me angry that you put me in this position of anxiety!") Imagine the impact on the employee's self esteem that this kind of termination has.

With some coaching, the supervisor might be able to use an alternative approach, saying, "You and I made a mistake in putting you in this job. I think we can both see this is not working out. I know that you are disappointed, as am I. However, this can be a learning experience for both of us. While this job is not right for you, I can see that you have a variety of skills that would be helpful in a number of jobs." It would still hurt to lose the job. However, under the second approach it is more easily experienced as a bad event, not a commentary on the rest of one's life. We can help these bad, uncomfortable events happen more humanely.

WHO IS THE CLIENT?

Sorting out who the client is may not be an easy task. That is true some-times in our traditional services as well. In People-Consulting in the Work-place a safe assumption is that the client is the one who pays your bill. We must serve our client's needs. If a company is paying, then the com-pany is your client. Your task is to serve the company's well-being. Be-fore getting too uncomfortable with that idea, keep reading.

As therapy has slipped deeper and deeper into managed care, it has become increasingly clear that managed care companies have become the clients, not the people sitting in our office. That is why it is so important to let go of third-party reimbursement.

What, then, about letting whole corporations become clients? What happens to the individual employees? This question speaks to the tradi-tion within our profession of being sensitive to power differentials and taking action when those less powerful seem to be getting hurt. This is a valid part of our tradition, but it can be overdone when it leads us to distort our perceptions of how things work.

For example, many young clinicians who work with children see them-selves as saviors of those children. There is an unconscious assumption that children need protection from their (diabolical) parents. Sometimes children do need protection, such as in situations of clear abuse. In most families, however, parents and children form systems in which they af-fect one another. As we learn to appreciate that children are not angels, and parents are not devils, greater maturity and helpfulness enter our services.

The same is true for work sites. There are some abusive employers. You are unlikely to be asked to provide services to companies in which employers are genuinely committed to abusiveness. If you stumble into such a situation and there is no hope of change, you will know that it is time to move on.

In most companies, as in most families, you will find a collection of well-meaning people, all of whom are flawed. Systems theory teaches us that each person in a system limits others, each helps others, and each has some measure of power, even if he or she *looks* small. One of the lessons of systems theory is that few people are truly powerless—it's just that people access power in different ways.

This perspective leads us to one of the major contributions that clini-cians can make. Systems theory helps support the new thinking in busi-ness that employee interests and company interests overlap far more than most people realized in the past. For too long, it was believed that the relationship between employer and worker *must* be adversarial. This be-lief has done great damage to both management and labor.

As I am writing this, a current news story comes out of Peoria, Illinois, about Caterpillar, Inc. A strike had lasted 17 months. Union members finally called it off because it was not getting them anywhere. The workers will get their jobs back. There is a belief that the company won. "I think the company's in complete control. We have to accept defeat," said one striker. Yet, we can safely predict that the powerful feelings that accompany that statement will find strong expression in work behaviors once people are back on the job. The company, overtly in complete control, is quite likely to pay the price for "winning."

As therapists, we are experts at finding and articulating overlapping interests. We do so whenever we are engaged in marital and family therapy. We are experts at finding ways to make seemingly competing interests compatible. Better than compromise, how many times, when working with couples, have you and your clients discovered solutions in which both parties can get what they seek? We can bring that perspective to People-Consulting in the Workplace.

This does not mean that all tension between management and workers will be eliminated. Their interests do not overlap 100%. However, that tension can be used creatively to solve problems. It does not have to be a reason for all-out warfare. Nor does it mean that therapists will be effective just using marital therapy techniques on labor/management issues. It is the win–win perspective that is being identified here.

The client is the *company,* not just management. The company is a collection of individuals, all of whom have a stake in the company's doing well. People may have different roles to play in the company, but what they share is some investment (albeit to different degrees) in the company's prosperity. Your job is to help the various groups within the company work toward outcomes that are good for *all* participants. We want to work toward win–win outcomes, because in any other outcome the one who wins will lose in the near future as the *process* of unproductive conflict continues. When that happens, the client (the company) did not get its money's worth from you.

A potential problem for you as the consultant in such situations is that, almost always, you have been hired by a member of the management team. Management usually has the role of making such decisions. We do need to keep decision makers happy in order to maintain our role (and income). However, this does not mean that we have to be their toadies. One CEO hired me as a general consultant to his company because I was willing to disagree with him and politely but firmly challenge his decisions. That kind of input is often difficult for CEOs to get from people whose entire incomes are based on their blessing.

You have been able to maintain your objectivity in the face of financial pressure before. If you treat children, do you always tell parents what they want to hear? When you do marital work, do you always side with the person who pays the bill? In fact, is taking sides even the issue? Even in individual therapy, we must give people negative feedback sometimes. Part of our skill is the ability to provide honest feedback conveying disturbing information in ways that enable the information to be useful to the recipient.

To be useful in our consultations to businesses, we must guard against our prejudices. We must guard against the temptation to give instant gratification to the person who sees to it that we get paid. We must also guard against temptations to side *automatically* with those we see as one-down (i.e., the weaker party).

> She was a therapist from New York City. She talked about the improvement of one of her long-term clients: "I'm sure what I did even helped her employer. Of course, I didn't mean to!"

Why not? What is wrong with helping employers? If we do it right, we will find ways that each participant can get something of value. In this situation the client was a therapy client, so of course that is where the therapist's allegiance belonged. But the wonderful thing is that, for the most part, we do not have to choose.

By helping companies improve their psychological working conditions, you can contribute tremendously to the financial well-being of the company. This helps employees to keep their jobs. In addition, your work can contribute to the emotional well-being of everyone in the company. In fact, that is the basic idea. Thus, employees often wind up working for a more profitable company, which enhances job security, and have a much more pleasant workplace in the bargain.

Part of our task is to bring communication where there has been polarization. We can bring understanding where there has been mistrust. We can help people to replace failure with success and incompetence with new skills. The opportunities to accomplish these things at work are limited only by our imagination.

Will we run into barriers? Sure. These are called resistances. We know all about them. We will find them in both employer and employee. They are a natural part of the processes of learning and changing. When we see resistances on the part of individuals whom we define as one down, we tend to be understanding. When we see resistances on the part of those we define as more powerful, something seems to erode that understanding. This blocks our ability to relate as a change agent with management, even when the changes we are trying to get them to make would help employees, as well.

He capriciously cut the bonus his executives counted on for income. This was the real-life version of *National Lampoon's Christmas Vacation* with Chevy Chase. In real life, it wasn't funny. This time, however, a clinician heading up a consultation project was able to help him see the error of his ways. No one else in the company was in a position to provide him this feedback. While the clinician was not gentle with him, she also did not alienate herself from him in moral outrage. That would have helped no one. The outcome was that the executives got their bonus.

To sum up my answer to the questions of who is the client and why is company money not third-party money, I would say that the company as a whole, with everybody in it, is the client. That means the people who receive your services and the people who pay the bill are one and the same. With third-party money, that is not the case.

BENEFITS FOR PARTICIPANTS IN PEOPLE-CONSULTING IN THE WORKPLACE

Three groups of people are involved in People-Consulting in the Workplace: employers, employees, and therapists. All benefit greatly:

- Employers' profits increase (which is why they would buy your services).
- Employees have better working conditions, more secure jobs, improved skills, and are happier with their own performance (which is why they would accept your services).
- You will make unmanaged money, advance your profession, and provide creative and satisfying applications of your skills (which is why you would offer these services).

People-Consulting in the Workplace is not a new idea. Relatively small numbers of clinicians have been doing it for decades. It is an exciting and rewarding field of great opportunity that is vastly underdeveloped.

BENEFITS FOR OUR PROFESSION AND OUR SOCIETY

It is important that more of us do People-Consulting in the Workplace because, by normalizing our services, so much is done to advance our profession. Normalizing our services will lead to an infinitely wider dissemination of our knowledge and skills than has been true to date. This increased dissemination of knowledge will do much to prevent a great many of the psychologically destructive behaviors and beliefs that currently create so much clinical repair work for us, and so much suffering for others.

How can People-Consulting in the Workplace help to accomplish this? Ask yourself this question: What is one hallmark that signals that people have taken their place in society as responsible adults? They go to work. Where, then, will we find people who are considered by society as being the most normal? At work. The people at work are functioning. Work takes up at least half of all waking adult hours. People put a lot of themselves into their jobs. They dress up; they try to be on their best behavior; and they measure their success by what happens on the job.

Of course, we know that many of the things that happen at work are not so good. That is why there are so many opportunities for us there. However, if we can make it normal for people like us to be hired by companies to help with those problems, imagine the impact on society's view of our services. What has just been for "crazy people" will now be acceptable for everyone. I look forward to the day when as many companies hire people like us as hire lawyers and accounting firms. When we approach human work issues with the Problem-Solving/Skill-Building model, rather than via psychopathology, shame barriers become eliminated, just as they do within traditional services.

Adding to the value of these services is the fact that many of them will be delivered to more than one person at a time. When in our offices, most of us still see one person at a time. With People-Consulting in the Workplace we will more often see people in groups, multiplying the impact of our services.

We are also likely to reach many more men this way, sometimes men who hold potentially powerful positions of social influence. Historically, men are more reluctant than women to start therapy, though, once they do, they tend to stay longer. Services like ours, offered as business training rather than "psychotherapy," will be much more palatable to them than in the past.

In addition, workers are likely to take personal skills learned in work-related training home. Because it is normal for people to discuss lessons from business training with their families, employees are more likely to share ideas at home. The lessons may then get extended to family relationships, whereas therapy lessons are sometimes kept secret.

He is an engineer in a shop full of engineers. He came home grumbling to his wife about this new trainer at work who was teaching engineers how to get along with each other. "This is stupid! It's a waste of time. We don't need it," he said. Several weeks later, as they were planning a family project, his wife nearly fainted when he suggested, "Shouldn't we include the kids in this discussion? You know, see how they feel about it?"

By meeting us on the job within normalized situations, a far greater percentage of the population will get to know us. This gives us a chance to wash away the prejudiced ideas that exist about who we are. Many people who first meet us through People-Consulting in the Workplace may later call us for traditional services. Indeed, clinicians who have done this work for several years tell me that it is a great way to generate referrals. Some of those referrals can be accepted directly because the nature of the services delivered on the job does not create conflicts of interest. Other times, referral to a colleague is appropriate. Either way, more work is getting generated. Your colleague may refer to you next time.

Finally, there is the issue of our own bottom line. We need to make money. Where is the money? In business. Remember that the role of business is the creation of wealth. Businesses are learning more and more that their biggest asset is their employees. The better trained employees are, both in terms of technical skills and people skills, the more productive they can be. The more productive they are, the greater is their value to the company.

Business people are not afraid to invest money when they believe it will improve their profits. In fact, they plan to invest certain amounts of their money in creating profit. Unlike some of us, they do not take every penny home with them at the end of the week. They save some to reinvest in the future. However, they need help from people like us to learn how People-Consulting in the Workplace can lead to improved profits.

ARE YOU QUALIFIED?

I found that many of the people offering psychologically oriented services to companies do not have our depth of training in human understanding. Some people seem to have picked up important knowledge elsewhere and provide value in their consultations. Others, however, are offering shallow services out of canned formulas.

> I happened to meet a man on an airplane who made his living helping companies motivate their employees. Though friendly enough with me, he was clearly such a disagreeable man that it strained my imagination to see him as effective. Yet he talked, convincingly, of a booming business. He had no training in psychology or any related field. He had a business background but apparently once had read a book on reinforcement theory. His understanding of human moti-

vation was terribly shallow. Yet, so few of us have offered our services to business that companies are vulnerable to using services such as he offered. Further, the psychological principles he invoked are so powerful that they can sometimes be helpful even when they are imperfectly articulated. Imagine how powerful they can be when laid out by knowledgeable professionals.

A psychologist once asked me if clinicians should do People-Consulting in the Workplace, given that the American Psychological Association (APA) has taken the stand that services to business and industry should be reserved for organizational/industrial psychologists. Actually, to my knowledge APA has not taken such a stand. In fact, during recent conversations with an executive with the Practice Directorate, it became clear to me that the APA is *supportive* of clinical psychologists engaging in appropriate forms of consultation to the business community. Yet, the question is central to concerns many of us have. We do not want to offer services we are unprepared to provide in a high quality manner. As long as we maintain that attitude, we will do well. What is important is distinguishing between the issues of titles and competence.

The APA ethical standards require that psychologists work within areas of competence, as developed by training and experience. Notice that the standard is not that we must have a Ph.D. in industrial psychology before offering any services whatsoever to the business community. Of course, before we use the *title* "industrial psychologist" we must have that Ph.D. and/or license. However, to work in the business community, the standard is whether we have prepared ourselves to do so.

Clinically trained professionals have been consulting to business about a wide range of issues for decades. Bob Rosen is one. Harry Levinson, Ph.D., is another psychologist who has made outstanding contributions to the business community. Levinson in particular makes the case that clinicians, with their understanding of individual issues, can provide great benefit to the expansion of business's ability to enhance its workforce. Saul Gellerman, Ph.D., whom we will meet shortly, is a third psychologist, originally trained as a clinician, who has made great contributions to the business world through his professional consultations.

The licensing law for clinical psychologists in Virginia specifically permits us to provide services such as I am labeling "People-Consulting in the Workplace." However, licensure, like a title, is not enough. My family physician is licensed to do brain surgery. Still, if I need some, I will find someone else, someone who has become competent in that area.

Experts in organizational development might criticize clinicians for not understanding organizational issues. Just as there is a wealth of information to be learned about clinical theory and practice, there is a body of literature that speaks to issues within organizational behavior. Depending on your goals, you will need to be more or less familiar with that literature. Reviewing possible services within People-Consulting in the Workplace (as in Chapter 10) shows that some projects will require more knowledge of organizational issues than others. The more that you do provide services that involve organizational issues, the more you will need to take steps to acquire the necessary knowledge and skills.

My experience within my clinical practice, which I suspect is representative of a large proportion of therapists, is that using a mix of individual and family systems ideas works well. Likewise, using our knowledge of individual issues combined with an appreciation of work systems issues will serve us well in People-Consulting in the Workplace. It is a powerful combination.

If you have developed an understanding of systems theory through working with families, you have already taken some important steps toward understanding organizations. Families and business systems are both alike and different in certain key ways. In terms of similarities:

• Families and companies are human groups with goals. This means that organized patterns of behavior will develop that guide individuals and the group as a whole. It is important to understand what goals the group has. Differences in goals lead to differences in behavioral norms.
• Interpersonal difficulties are a given in both family and business groups. Just as every human being has difficulties in living, so does every family and business. No two human beings ever have identical needs, goals, or styles.
• Communications, hierarchy, and boundary issues are always present in human groups, whether at home or at work. These are fundamental concerns that every group must handle.
• Much of what people learn about operating in groups is learned in their family of origin. As clinicians know, this learning often becomes unconscious, because much of it was learned at an age when lessons go fundamentally unquestioned.

However, these similarities do not give us permission just to carry our ways of doing clinical work over to the job site, lock, stock, and barrel. Adaptations must be made or we will fail and look silly doing it. Some adaptations are related to how families and business groups are different:

• Families and groups have different reasons for existing. We sometimes get confused about this, getting upset when employers do not give their employees the same unconditional positive regard families are supposed to give. Businesses have also gotten confused on this point some-times, saying: "We are just one big happy family." Employees often roll their eyes when they hear statements like this. The truth is that com-panies make poor families because that is not what they are supposed to be.

The distinction between work and home can best be understood by recalling how people develop self-esteem. Self-esteem has two sources: who loves and likes us, and what we are good at. It is the job of the fam-ily to offer the nurturance and unconditional positive regard people need to build that side of their self-esteem. The role of an employer is to give the employee an opportunity to make a living, within which he can de-velop and use skills, which will feed the other side of self-esteem. Love at work is unlikely and unnecessary. Respect, liking, and sometimes af-fection can all arise. However, even these feelings will be lost if the em-ployer or employee is incompetent. In addition, Noer, in *Healing the Wound* (1993), points out that when businesses try to create too much of a family atmosphere, employees often become overly dependent upon their employer. This interferes with the employees' performance and creativity.

Therefore, do not enter People-Consulting in the Workplace with romantic notions about what the emotional context of the workplace should be. A positive emotional context certainly enhances performance. Performance, however, is the fundamental issue in a workplace setting.

• Because families and businesses have different reasons for exist-ing, there are different behavioral expectations for people within each. As you go about your consultations, be clear about what appropriate ex-pectations are.

• Different emotional connections develop between family members than develop among workmates. Consider what happens when this rule is violated. When a romance develops in the office, it creates tremendous disruption. Coworkers get upset; work becomes confused. This kind of relationship does not belong at work. Thus, when you work as a consul-tant with a company, respect the appropriate differences in emotional con-nections between family members and workmates. Otherwise, you may attempt to facilitate a degree of connection and intimacy that interfers with the fundamental task and well-being of the organization. When that hap-pens, everybody loses.

• Finally, we can take the transference hypothesis only so far. While much of how we learn to behave does come from our family of origin, the immediate situation is also a powerful determiner of behavior. If some-one hates his boss, it may be because the boss is really behaving badly, not because of unfinished authority figure business. If a boss is angry with an employee, transference issues may be irrelevant. It may be that the employee habitually behaves irresponsibly.

WHAT TRAINING DO I NEED?

Of course, the answer to this question is "It depends." None of us will have such wide-ranging competencies that we will be able to provide every service that might fall under People-Consulting in the Workplace, just as no clinician offers every possible clinical service. Thus, as you choose the areas you want to pursue, you will either want to select issues that fit your knowledge or build your knowledge to fit areas of interest to you.

For example, if you have practiced psychoanalytic therapy with individuals for 20 years, you probably are not prepared to provide independent consultation around corporate cultural change. However, doing a combination of reading and carefully selected workshops is likely to build on your base of skills. Having more experienced consultants available for consultation is extremely useful, as well.

Alternatively, many clinicians are likely to find it a short transition from their normal work to such services as setting up a trauma response plan, executive coaching, many aspects of conflict management training, self-esteem development, health promotion programs, and coaching interpersonal skills for supervisors. Even with these, though, an appreciation of how work and personal lives differ will be important. Do what you would do if you moved to a foreign country: Learn the culture and the issues.

Part of my message is that as a clinician you are far more ready for this work than you may realize. Remember that basically we are talking about applying the Problem-Solving/Skill-Building model at work. However, the workplace does offer enough uniqueness to make it worth your while to consider what additional training or reading or experience would be useful to you.

No amount of preparation will *fully* prepare you for this field. Similarly, no amount of preparation prepares us *fully* to do therapy. We have chosen jobs in which it is impossible to know all there is to know, much less know what remains to be discovered. Professionals get paid for making judgments. This means we usually have to operate with some measure of doubt. People who follow rigid recipes based on all the facts are called technicians.

People sometimes use not knowing everything as an excuse for inaction. Therapists, legislative bodies, committees, and businesses all dodge tough issues by waiting for more study. Imagine if people waited until they "knew enough" before getting married or having children. It would pretty much take care of the population explosion.

Of course, people are sometimes too impulsive (though this is out of character for most therapists, who love to ponder issues instead of taking action). A certain amount of preparation is appropriate before beginning. How much and what kind of preparation you need will depend on your experiences and what services you choose to offer. First, do an analysis of what you already know and then see what gaps remain.

A Skills Assessment

Let's begin determining your needs by doing a skills assessment. Consider how the following experiences, many of which you have had, prepare you for People-Consulting in the Workplace.

Are you trained and experienced in group therapy? If the answer is yes, you understand how to observe group process. This is an extremely valuable skill to have when doing business training. In business training, you are not a college professor presenting material that students had better learn. Rather, through your training, you goal is to be a *change agent.* Group therapy experiences help you know how to bring a group together. You know how to offer safe experiential exercises and how to handle the strong affect that sometimes arises within group settings. You know how to read the mood of the group, watching for level of interest and opportunities for emotional change. You know how to read the signs that people are running into resistances, which will happen in 100% of your training experiences. All of these skills are valuable when facilitating work groups in problem solving or team building.

However, the goals of work-based training are different from the goals of group therapy, and the relationships between the participants are different, as well. Keep that in mind.

I was a 3rd-year graduate student doing a practicum at the University Counseling Center. The faculty/staff was a group of talented therapists who, for the most part, were also fine human beings. They decided to use their skills to help their own work relationships. They met once a week, trying to use encounter techniques (this was in the early 1970s). As a student, I was not invited, so I cannot give a first-hand report. However, the unanimous decision, after a few months, was to give this up as a bad idea. Their discovery was that, as a work group, they had different goals than therapy groups and thus needed to approach their interpersonal issues differently.

If *this* group could not make a group therapy model work, I feel quite confident that others cannot, as well. However, some aspects of those skills appear to be quite useful in certain kinds of training experiences. It is a matter of fitting the technique to the purposes and realities of the participants.

Are you trained and experienced with family systems? If yes, you know something about how systems work. Mastering the ability to think in a systemic way is invaluable to understanding work groups, which, of course, also function in systems. Someone who knows systems can bring a much greater depth of understanding to work situations than those still stuck in linear thinking. You know, for example, that linear thinking often promotes the search for scapegoats. While sometimes there really are bad actors, a systems approach permits a much wider choice of possible explanations of the problems. You can learn how to help companies differentiate culture or systems-based problems from individual-based problems.

Have you ever been employed by an organization? If you have, you have personally experienced organizational dynamics, though you may have called it politics. If you kept your eyes open, you could observe how group and individual issues interacted. You knew what it was like to be on the receiving end sometimes. If you had a leadership position, you know it provided less power than you thought it would when you accepted it. You could become aware of how groups and forces external to the organization also had an impact on life within the organization.

Have you ever done emergency crisis counseling? Then you have experience that can help you to assist a company in setting up a crisis response team (see Chapter 10). Having dealt with therapy clients in emotional crisis gives you a feeling for the emotional intensity involved. If you have done actual trauma work, so much the better. The corporate CEO and the Vice President for Human Relations are unlikely to have had such experiences.

Have you ever helped an executive change? If you have ever had a client who happened to be an executive and if the two of you ever considered work issues, then you have done many aspects of executive coaching. You know something about the issues and processes involved. If you now enter this process by being retained by an employer, you may gain increased perspective on how things look both from an executive's side and from the company's.

Have you ever consulted with schools or agencies about services and problem solving? If so, you have gotten outside the comfort of your office. This is a good move. Also, you have experience dealing with organizations. You know that it is a challenging process, with many threads to keep track of. You know that they sometimes throw consultants their most difficult (usually impossible) situation as a test.

Have you ever run a business, even if only your own private prac-

tice? If so, then you already know something about how it feels to be in business. You have dealt with the issues of profit and loss and meeting expenses. You know something about the risk involved and the wish for success. You know something about keeping books and perhaps supervising personnel. Such experiences can help you identify with the issues and concerns of company leaders.

Usually, during my seminar, as I ask these questions, most hands shoot up as "yes" to each question. The participants had not previously realized how relevant these experiences are to People-Consulting in the Workplace. As they realize that many of their professional and life experiences have helped prepare them for this new work, and as they see how many of the potential services are extensions of things they have already done, optimism begins to develop.

The next step in evaluating your training needs is to look further into your background to see what you already have done. Since I cannot know what is in your background, I will share with you the process I went through evaluating my own background for People-Consulting in the Workplace. I was then, not so long ago, where you may be now. By looking at how some of my experiences were relevant, I hope you will see how your experiences may be applicable.

University Training

In the early 1970s, when I attended Florida State for my doctorate in clinical psychology, community psychology was a hot topic. We took classes and seminars that helped us learn about group functioning and consulting to organizations. As a student project, we set up a crisis counseling line as a part of the University Counseling Center. That forced us to look at the impact of this service on the community, training issues, and how housing this service impacted upon the Counseling Center itself. Perhaps you have experiences from your training that are similar.

Seminars

Several seminars have been extremely helpful. Two of the best, "Organizational Development" and "Facilitating Organizational Change," were offered by University Associates (see the Appendix). Participants were a mix of business people employed by corporations and therapists broadening their skills. Leaders were business consultants who teach these workshops on the side. We learned some important theoretical material in relatively painless ways. Much of it built easily on the foundation provided by our psychological training and experiences. At the same time, we could learn about business culture from the business participants, and we could learn about business consulting from the leaders.

Rodney Lowman, Ph.D., has offered a one-day workshop on executive assessment, oriented toward helping companies pick the best candidate for executive positions. Business psychologists tell me that this is a well-accepted way to begin a relationship with a company. Lowman's course offered an excellent theoretical model and tools that are readily useful to someone with a solid background in assessment. In addition, this workshop was also useful in getting a look inside the world of business, learning about executives' key issues and needs.

About 12 years ago, my partner and I took a workshop on developing and selling EAPs, back in the days when we thought we wanted to be in the EAP business. We eventually decided it was not for us. Still, the seminar was another window into the world of business. Having the seminar in my background helps me understand the difference between EAPs and People-Consulting in the Workplace. It helps me to relate knowledgeably to the EAP person in a business where I may be interested in doing a project.

As we were getting ready to open Peak Performance Consultation, my partner and I, accompanied by a few other brave souls who were volunteers in the Virginia Marketing Project, took a one-day sales course with the president of a company that specializes in sales training. It was extremely valuable, teaching us that sales and therapy have more in common than we ever dreamed. It helped reduce our anxiety level and again gave us a window into the business community.

Finally, just recently, four of us arranged a day-long private consultation with Saul Gellerman, Ph.D. Dr. Gellerman was trained as a clinical psychologist but early on decided he preferred working within business. He began with a company that tested executive job candidates. Then he worked for IBM and later became an independent consultant to major companies all over the world. He now is on the business faculty of the University of Dallas, recently stepping down from 8 years as the Dean of the Business School. His input was extremely useful in adding to our understanding of how to approach various business-related psychological problems.

The story of how this consultation was arranged may be of interest to you. We had noticed that Dr. Gellerman was offering a workshop in St. Lucia that looked really useful. It was an appealing idea, taking the workshop in the morning and then sunning in the Caribbean in the afternoon. However, when we began to add up the cost of the workshop, travel, meals, hotel, and being out of the office, it got very expensive. We realized that, with a few people chipping in, it would be much cheaper to pay him a sizable consulting fee and his expenses and bring him to us. In fact, we saved 60%.

What workshops have you taken over the years? Which ones could you take now to build on the skills that you have been acquiring over the course of your career? Who do you know that you could call on for consultation?

Experiences

Over the past 22 years, I have taken advantage of a number of opportunities that, in retrospect, have been extremely helpful in getting me ready for People-Consulting in the Workplace. I suspect that many of your experiences have also been adding to your preparation.

As an employee early in my career, I functioned within both a community mental health center and later a large private psychiatric hospital. These experiences helped me learn about politics and organizational dynamics. Did you ever work in such places? What about your graduate training program—were there any internal politics there?

With regard to trauma work, I had the chance to work with two sets of bank employees who had just experienced holdups at gunpoint, an experience that will be detailed in the next chapter. Several of us in the Manassas Group serve on the crisis team for a local high school. This has led to a number of sad but important experiences in helping students cope with the sudden deaths of friends and classmates.

In 1979, I was asked to do a psychological evaluation on a troubled employee of a local company. The CEO liked my report and asked for an evaluation on another employee. When that one was finished, he asked me to develop an EAP. In fact, this was to become the first EAP in the Roanoke Valley. Developing that program required consideration of a variety of organizational issues.

Over the years, I have been called on to lead a variety of training events in the community. These included setting up a program for people to work with child-abusive parents and helping a broad range of professionals learn about responding to suicidal issues of adolescents.

Finally, my role in conceptualizing and implementing the Virginia Marketing Project for the Virginia Academy of Clinical Psychologists (VACP) was a great experience in dealing with organizational issues. Such issues exist within VACP, just as they do in every other organization. We dealt with politics, resistance to change, external forces, and a host of other issues that come up in People-Consulting in the Workplace.

Reading

In addition to these experience, there are many good written resources available. My bookshelves now contain a great many books that have been useful in broadening my understanding of the business world and its issues. In the Appendix, you will find a wide variety of resources that have been useful in developing the entire program presented in this book. Among those resources are some of the best of the business oriented books.

OTHER QUESTIONS

How are we doing in handling your questions? Our seminar participants usually ask a number of questions that might be sorted under the title "miscellaneous" and yet are important.

Where will I get the energy? Of course, it depends on your own personality makeup. However, many people find that, as they move into a new area, the process of creativity generates new energy. It is exciting to see that you can develop new skills and apply old skills in new ways. That energy is likely to spread back into other areas of your practice. It has in mine.

Will I have anything of value to offer? Yes. Actually, I hope this has been answered already.

I don't know the language. Read some of the books offered in the Appendix. Check the bookstore for titles that help people learn about business etiquette. Saul Gellerman encouraged us to take an accounting class or a business management class. Not only would you learn some useful skills but you would also learn about the language of business. Talk with some business people. Perhaps you have friends and relatives in the business world. Renew those relationships. Most people, especially relatives, are thrilled to give advice.

I am an introvert. Do I have the personality for this? This is like therapy. It is such a broad area that it has room for a broad range of personality styles. One participant in a recent conference told us: "I am an introvert. I do a lot of executive coaching. It works for me."

Will businessmen and -women take us seriously? They will if you have a way to convince them that you can help their company's productivity. The next three chapters should help you to develop that argument. They will also take you seriously if you do not act "weird." Business people have prejudiced ideas about us, just as we do about them. They see us as weird. Some of our colleagues help to reinforce that image by, among other things: being exceedingly verbose, seeming overly intellectual rather than practical, acting pompous, portraying a goody-goody image that seems inconsistent with the real world, and dressing like an absent-minded professor rather than in business attire.

Can women succeed at this, or is this a man's game? As a man, I am short of personal experience from which to answer this question. However, I have known and know of a number of women who have done well in People-Consulting in the Workplace. Two are the women who run Creative Dimensions in Management. If you are a psychologist, you may have seen their workshop ads in the *APA Monitor*. Their business consulting is focused on helping companies to implement culture change by means of therapy with the leading executives.

Another woman who reports success specializes in helping companies set up trauma response plans. She told me that that service constitutes about 40% of her billable time, with the remainder given over to traditional clinical work.

Recently, I attended a presentation at *The Family Therapy Networker* Symposium by Ilene Wasserman, M.S.W., on the application of family therapy skills to business consultation. She did not discuss this specific issue, but I doubt that anyone in the room left feeling that women could not do this type of work. Nor did they see any evidence that femininity must be sacrificed in order to do it well. What seems to matter is a sense of confidence, of competence, and of genuineness.

A participant in our seminar in Maine was a business psychologist whose purpose in coming to our seminar was to learn more about clinical work. He reported that his firm frequently assigned women consultants to companies led by highly competitive men. They found that these men could often put their competitive agendas aside when dealing with women, allowing their softer sides to show.

It is possible that these women were more accepted as consultants than they would have been if they actually worked as employees in the firm. This is because, while a lot of the permanent upper level executive slots still seem to be reserved for men, many companies will readily use women consultants, such as attorneys, physicians, and accountants.

Sometimes this question about women in consulting is asked by people with a particular kind of business executive in mind. The stereotypical picture is usually that of a gruff, macho, "no-nonsense," insensitive, Type-A man. There are executives like him. However, there are many other kinds of business people, too, of both sexes. Just as you work with certain personality types better than with other types in therapy, you will find that you are more accepted by some business personality types than others. No one holds all the cards. What is an advantage in one situation is a disadvantage in another.

One of the most valuable experiences I have had in preparing myself for this work has been asking for information and opinions from others. If I were a woman interested in breaking into this area, I would spend some time talking with women who have been successful in the business world. While sexism certainly exists, some women find ways to do well. Find out what they know and use it to turn the odds in your favor.

SUMMARY

People-Consulting in the Workplace is the application of the Problem-Solving/Skill-Building model to problems in the workplace. All people struggle with developing the optimal psychological skills for their jobs, and all jobs involve problem solving. Understanding that this is a universal need frees us from having to box people into arbitrary categories before offering services. It is not just about the bad things (symptoms) that can happen. It is also about the good things that do not happen when people are not at their best. Everybody involved benefits.

We have looked at a number of questions therapists often have in terms of ethics, training, and other concerns about doing People-Consulting in the Workplace. Hopefully, we will continue to cross questions off your list as we deal, in the next three chapters, with the nitty-gritty of getting started.

Chapter 10

Learning from Those in the Workplace and Where That Can Lead

THE MORPHING OF A CLINICIAN

We have been discussing the shift that can be made by a full-time clinician, with valuable skills to sell to the community, into a part-time consultant, with valuable skills to sell to business. In my own case, two additional exposures to the business community helped me envision the contributions that clinicians can make to the well-being of employers and employees.

LESSONS FROM THE VIRGINIA MARKETING PROJECT

Between 1992 and 1995, I was involved in developing and administering the Virginia Marketing Project for the Virginia Academy of Clinical Psychologists (VACP). As a part of that program, VACP commissioned our marketing consultant, Frank Taylor, to do a market study of employers. The study allowed us to hear from the business community about their perceptions of us and their possible needs. The results of this study were a cornerstone in the conceptualization of "People-Consulting in the Workplace."

The original goal of the Virginia Marketing Project was to create relationships with employers so that we could educate them about the value of outpatient therapy. As discussed in Part I, we hoped that this would lead them to adjust their outpatient mental health benefits to align with our beliefs about good clinical service. While we did not achieve that goal, we achieved something I believe to be better. We learned that there are many behavior-based, not pathology based, services that we could provide to business. This learning helped awaken me to the immense opportunities available to therapists in the workplace.

For the market study, Frank visited 36 major employers in Virginia, spending 45 minutes with the decision maker on health care benefits, doing a semistructured interview. The companies ranged in size from 400 to 80,000 employees. Ten industries were represented, as were a variety of types of ownership, that is, publicly held companies, privately held companies, government entities, etc. We looked at three areas: (1) worker productivity, (2) psychologically oriented services business wants, and (3) health care benefits related to outpatient therapy. For our present purposes, results from the first two areas are presented.

Worker Productivity

The goal of every business is to make a profit. As reported in Chapter 9, a major key to profit is worker productivity. If a company succeeds in raising its productivity by even 1%, profit can respond dramatically. Productivity is related more to psychological issues than the business community has historically realized. Bob Rosen's book *The Healthy Company* (1991) helps us, and them, see that. We wanted to know what Virginia business people were thinking in this area so that we could better know how to approach them.

The vast majority of employers dealt with our questions about productivity in the same way. They reported that (1) their productivity is "normal," (2) the productivity of other businesses in the state is below normal, and (3) their own productivity "could be better." What do these three statements mean when taken together? It is a safe assumption that all companies worry about productivity; yet, it is a sensitive area. Perhaps it was difficult for participants to admit significant productivity problems to a stranger. Businesses, however, could speak indirectly about such problems through their comments about other companies and by expressing their belief that their own productivity could be improved.

What factors seem to impair productivity? Participants outlined a number of psychologically based issues:

- Downsizings are rampant in business today, resulting in employee insecurity. This, in turn, often leads to "malicious obedience." In other words, employees do *exactly* what they are told—and no more. Employees who totally suspend their own judgement are not highly productive.

- Many managers are seen as having poor interpersonal skills. This is the oft-told tale about individuals gaining promotions on the basis of good technical skills. These skills are usually unrelated to the interpersonal skills required to create and lead a productive work group.
- Companies are not spending enough time or money on training their employees. This is especially interesting given that employers also complained that young people now entering the workforce bring a disappointing set of skills.
- Only 50% of employers identified family stresses as creating productivity problems. This shows we have not done well communicating what we know to be true about the relationship between family stress and work life.
- Only 25% of employers recognized that psychological problems affect physical health. They were, of course, aware that physical health problems constrain productivity. We have failed to communicate what we know about where much of that physical illness comes from.
- We had expected that absenteeism would be a concern. Yet, only one-third of companies complained about an absenteeism problem. A major reason for this finding, however, was that most of the companies had not figured out how to measure absenteeism. (Those of you with a research background can probably think of many ways *that* problem could be solved.)

Psychologically Oriented Services Business Wants

With a little imagination, you can begin to see that you are, or can easily become, knowledgeable in the areas employers identified as relevant to productivity problems. You can then begin to generate ideas about services we might offer. To seed this process with employers, Frank asked about specific areas of possible service. The results included:

- *Managers' interpersonal skills.* All participants but one wanted help in improving the relationship skills of managers. This concern is based on wanting to move from a *management model* to a *leadership model,* a hot topic in business today. It is a good example of how the business culture is changing in ways that create opportunities for people with our skills. Management is defined as what one can coerce others to do. Leadership is defined as winning the hearts and minds of those who follow. The potential productivity differences between these two models are obvious. Making the transition from management to leadership requires managers to change their attitudes and behaviors. Helping people to change attitudes and behaviors is our bread and butter.

- *Conflict on the job.* Conflict exists in all human organizations. Whenever you get even two people together for any extended period of time, some conflicts will arise. Therefore, conflict within any work organization is a given. Over 80% of the employers in our study were dissatisfied with how conflict within their own company was handled. Again, this is something we can help with. We know about interpersonal conflict; unlike most people, we are not frightened by the intense affect often associated with conflict, and we know how to lead conflict toward productive outcomes.

AN INVITATION TO CONSULT

Some time after the project was completed I received a phone call from Frank. "Dana, what do you know about downsizing? How do employees react?" he asked. He had talked with an executive in a large company that was going through a severe downsizing. Perhaps there was a consulting opportunity.

"Let me get back to you," I said. Downsizing in and of itself was not an area of expertise for me. But Frank was not suggesting that I consult about the financial aspects of downsizing. He was suggesting that there were psychological components of downsizing that would have a powerful impact on the process itself. His own experience as a leading executive within a large corporation told him that this was true. Further, evidence to support this idea had surfaced in the market study he had done for VACP. Since I did feel I knew something about psychological processes, I set out to see how much of what I already knew might be applicable.

We have a history of doing our homework. We do not get through graduate training without that skill. I began my homework in the form of a literature review. I found some good psychological research on what happens to survivors of downsizings, those who keep their jobs. The research shows that several factors influence how survivors respond both psychologically and behaviorally. The most powerful factor in determining employee reaction is the way in which the downsizing is handled by company leadership. Interestingly, this is also the most powerful factor in determining whether the downsizing will lead to financial improvement or financial disaster for the company.

In some downsizing companies, leaders seem to throw people out callously. An employee, with several years' tenure, a mortgage on his house, and all the trappings of a middle-class lifestyle, might be called in to his supervisor's office peremptorily and leave with instructions to clean out his desk and be gone within 30 minutes. A security guard might "help" ensure that the instructions are carried out. This person is a casualty of the downsizing.

Survivors are those who watch as friends and coworkers become casualties. Survivors respond to the observed inhumanity with anger, anxiety, and risk aversion. They become enraged that the company could be so disloyal and unfeeling. Survivors wonder if or when it will happen to them. In an attempt to avoid becoming a casualty, they play it safe, becoming maliciously obedient. Their malicious obediance is not only a response to their anxiety but also gives them a passive–aggressive outlet for the rage they experience.

Strong feelings are always expressed, one way or another. Survivors' feelings get expressed in their work. While downsizing companies need employees to work harder and more creatively than ever, survivors are too afraid and too angry to do so. Unintentionally, the leaders have established a culture of disloyalty at a time when loyalty is most critical to the company's success. No wonder that, despite the current popularity of downsizings in corporate America, business studies find that most downsizings fail to save money (Marshall, 1993).

David Noer is a business consultant and the author of *Healing the Wound* (1993), a book about how businesses can heal the wounds created by downsizings. Noer observed the emotional devastation created by insensitively handled "right sizings." He then figured out why leaders create such devastation. His consultation experiences taught him that company leaders who conduct downsizings in unfeeling ways are people who are isolated from their own feelings about the process. It is not, usually, that they are uncaring. They just do not know what to do with their feelings, so they ignore them.

Noer reasoned that, if leaders could be helped to understand their feelings and then given ways to show those feelings appropriately, the downsizing process might be handled better. He devised some methods that were useful within some of the situations he confronted. Noer describes what in other settings might be considered a therapeutic task—putting people in touch with their feelings and helping them to devise better ways of dealing with the trauma. That sounded like a familiar activity to me. Like most of you, I have made a career out of helping people to get in touch with their feelings and then find appropriate and effective ways to express them.

I would *like* to report that Frank and I did a bang-up consultation job with that downsizing company he talked to—but, unfortunately, we did not get hired for that project. Like our clinical clients, companies do not always do what we want them to do.

Lessons learned. The results of the VACP Market Study and my research on downsizing convinced me that our skills are applicable in environments other than our offices and that the resources are there to help us make the transition. When we redefine ourselves as agents of human change rather than as "mental illness treaters," we find that a variety of diversifications suddenly become available. If you look at your practice, you may see that it is not such a big step from the clinical world to the world of business consultation.

> This 16-year-old former honors student did not really want to fail his junior year of high school. However, he was enraged by his father's affair. At the time I met him, he knew no better way to express his rage. Expressing rage became more important than academic success. Our job was to develop better strategies to achieve both of his goals.

How is this adolescent's response to disloyalty different from that of the angry survivor of downsizing who engages in malicious obedience? Both people express anger toward an authority figure in passive ways that hit the mark but also seriously damage the expresser. Both are out of touch with their feelings and behave in ways that are intended to obscure the meaning of their behavior both from themselves and from the targets of their behavior. Why label one reaction a mental illness (Adjustment Reaction of Adolescence) and not the other? Actually, why label either one in a shame-based way?

There is usually a veritable army of angry, acting-out employees within downsizing companies. Why wait for them to wander into our offices by ones and twos? Why not offer services that can speak to the needs of the entire group (secondary prevention) or even offer services to business leaders that could avoid the whole mess (primary prevention)?

We know a lot about helping people get in touch with their feelings, just as company leaders who must downsize need to do. We know a lot about helping people, in this case company leaders, see the self-interest served by coming to terms with their feelings. We know a lot about helping people figure out how to handle and communicate feelings in productive ways. Experience tells me that almost everyone prefers mature emotional expression to denial and avoidance. They just need help sometimes figuring out how to achieve it.

Downsizing is representative of a number of workplace issues that I have now researched. My research involved reviewing literature, taking workshops, and talking with people involved in the process. As I did these things, clinical experience, combined with a modicum of imagination, led me to conceptualize ways that I could modify what I knew to make it serve the needs of the workplace. I believe that you will find that you can, too.

SERVICES THAT BUSINESS NEEDS

As outlined in Chapter 9, People-Consulting in the Workplace is the application of the Problem-Solving/Skill-Building model to the human issues within the workplace that interfere with people's feeling and doing their best on the job. We can bring this definition to life by delineating some of the many services that can fall under this rubric. This discussion is *not* intended to be exhaustive. It *is* intended to stimulate your imagination—to help you to figure out how what you already know, or can learn with relative ease, can be used to help people at work.

Conflict Management

Conflict management services are a natural fit with our skills, and the need exists. Remember that the VACP Marketing Study told us that 81% of companies are dissatisfied with how internal conflict is handled. How surprising should that be? Our society does a poor job of teaching conflict management skills. Some people are lucky enough to have good role models, but many, perhaps most, do not.

Ignorance about conflict management skills combines with the law of human behavior that says "When you don't know what to do, you do what you know." People who do not know good conflict management skills know avoidance. As a result, too many people in conflict with others avoid dealing with it openly. As experts, we know that conflict that gets avoided now will only resurface later, often in a disguised form.

Sometimes it is not so disguised. A 1993 Reuters report said that more than 2 million people had been physically attacked on the job during the preceding year. One in 6 had been attacked with a deadly weapon. Some 750 people had been murdered. Employers paid $4.2 billion to cover the costs of workplace violence.

The fact that conflict in the workplace is a problem is beginning to be acknowledged in the popular press. On July 4, 1993, a news article by Julie Gravelle appeared in the *Roanoke Times* with the headline "Conflicts among Workers Found to Hurt Bottom Line." Problems were said to stem from a variety of sources, including lack of assertiveness and poor decision making by leaders, as well as "an atmosphere of discontent" (p. F3).

If you do marital and family therapy, no one knows more about helping people deal with emotionally intense conflict than you do. Therapy provides a great training ground for dealing with the intense feelings often associated with conflict. Whereas most people in business, and most business consultants, are put off and frightened by intense affect, it is our bread and butter. We are comfortable in its presence, and we know how to handle it safely. We are skilled in helping people talk about issues that others avoid. Talking about these issues frees conflicted people to find their common interests.

This does not mean that we automatically know everything there is to know about *workplace* conflicts. Workplace conflicts and family conflicts differ in some ways. Just as family dynamics may be important variables in personal conflicts, organizational dynamics may play a role in workplace conflicts. General systems theory is extremely helpful here, just as family systems theory is helpful in understanding family conflict. However, *intense* conflicts are generally about human issues, and it is those issues upon which we base our expertise.

An old acquaintance thought he could use our services. He had set up his company from scratch. He was an energetic and persuasive man who won customers with his personality and kept them with excellent service. His Achilles heel, by his own admission, was his lack of organizational structure, and department heads fought one another viciously in unsuccessful efforts to establish a permanent pecking order.

A number-two man was hired to straighten things out, but he was not on the job long before he too was swept up in the conflict. The CEO's competitive nature just could not let the new man succeed where he himself had failed, and so he let the department heads eat his new assistant alive.

Our intervention began with interviews of all the key players—the CEO, his number-two man, and the department heads. Some line employees wanted to talk to us too. The ground rules we established were that we would share all information we deemed important, first in feedback sessions with the CEO and later in meetings with the department heads. We would not, however, reveal the sources of the comments.

What were the human issues? There were at least three. (1) All of these people wanted to have some control over their environment. Power is always an issue in human relationships. and unsettled power issues often lead to conflict. The lack of organization led people to use chaotic methods to gain control over their environment. These strategies worked well in the short run but had predictably negative long-term effects. (2) Self-esteem issues also got raised because conflicts led to accusations regarding the quality of work people were doing. (3) Communication issues were prominent. Few effective communication patterns had been established because there was no effective organizational structure and because communication would have brought too many things out in the open that people were trying to hide.

We learned that we were not the first consultants our friend had called in. Three business consultants had preceded us and all had failed. The staff was pessimistic about our making a difference. Yet, we did. We succeeded at helping the CEO and others in the company understand the issues and change their behaviors. We helped the group develop organizational structures and communication patterns that have worked for them.

Why did we succeed where others had failed? There were two reasons. First, we could get people to talk about some aspects of the relevant issues that preceding consultants could not. Therapists are experts in getting people to talk about difficult issues. We are also good at seeing symptoms as an attempt to solve a poorly understood problem, not the problem itself. Second, we knew how to feed the information back constructively, in ways everyone could use. Therapists are experts in helping people use information about themselves in new ways.

Leadership Training

As we discussed, VACP's Marketing Study found that business wants to move from a management model to a leadership model. It wants its leaders to be able to win the hearts and minds of their employees. Reading the business literature indicates that this is true nationwide.

This change requires potential leaders to connect with people in skillful, interpersonal ways, forming authentic relationships. Authentic relationships are essential building blocks of effective leadership. We know a lot about establishing authentic relationships. We know a lot about helping people behave in authentic ways. Business wants its leaders to change their attitudes and behaviors. We know a lot about helping people change attitudes and behaviors.

If you are like me, however, you may wonder about your own content knowledge of leadership itself. There are many good resources that can give you the content.

For example, Hogan, Curphy, and Hogan (1994) present a wonderful review of the psychological literature on leadership. It turns out that a highly useful body of research exists. The authors complain that it is woefully underutilized by psychologists. Reading their article will bring you up to speed on the literature.

Then, there are a number of excellent books on leadership written by and for the business community that you will find helpful. For example, John O'Neill, president of the California School of Professional Psychology, wrote *The Paradox of Success* (1993), which discusses leadership from a Jungian point of view. It succeeds extremely well in making the often difficult concepts Jung developed understandable to the psychological layman. Kouzes and Posner wrote *The Leadership Challenge* (1987), as well as a program for training leaders offered by Pfeiffer & Company (see the Appendix). While you may customize any prestructured program you buy, you usually do not have to reinvent the wheel. Finally, review your own experiences of leading and being led to help sensitize you to critical issues.

> After 27 years, he became president of the company. He had earned it. He examined his options of how to lead the company and asked good questions. The company culture had been highly autocratic, though beginning to soften in recent years. Still, he could see that autocratic behavior wending its way through the company, coming out, for example, in supervisory behavior that was often insensitive.
>
> Of course, after 27 years in this culture, he too had been affected. He knew that he did not want his supervisors acting this way but sometimes failed to catch himself being overly directive. He wanted to change some of the structure of the company, moving toward involving others in decision making (but he did not always see when he himself had been preventing that from happening).
>
> The original request for consultation involved the supervisors. As more information was developed, the methods whereby company leadership unintentionally maintained the undesirable behavior became evident. Also evident were the sincere interests of leaders to change their own behavior.
>
> The next stage of the consultation helped the top management team look at themselves and decide how they wanted to change. Each team member took a look at himself. They were as willing as any client—in other words, ambivalent. However, none of them maintained autocratic behaviors in isolation. They came to recognize that they were members/leaders of a system. The consultation task involved helping not just the president to change, but those around him, as well.

Stress Management Seminars

This is not what you would call a brand-new idea. Yet, these seminars continue to sell well and may be the easiest way to make an initial connection with a company. Having been around so long, they have become normalized, in that way making them easier to sell.

I had an opportunity in March 1995 to talk with Ronald Finch, former Vice President for Human Resources at BellSouth. It was Finch who worked with the APA to help them develop their Integrated Care Program. Finch is one executive who clearly values psychological services. His attitude proved to be financially beneficial to BellSouth in that the company literally saved a fortune with Integrated Care.

Over lunch he told me that, in 1985, he wanted 20,000 (20,000!)

of BellSouth's executives to take stress management training. He was willing to pay psychologists $1,000 per day (1985 dollars) to provide the service, but he could not find enough of them interested in doing it. Where were we!?

Toxic Stress Seminars

My partner and I wanted to differentiate ourselves from lesser trained competitors. We came up with Toxic Stress Management as an urgent issue of concern. Our plan is to offer the standard stress management fare but add to it from our depth of understanding as therapists.

Toxic Stress Management mixes a variety of elements and goals:

- We can focus on the interaction between work and home stress. We know from the Virginia Marketing Project that many business people have little appreciation for this interaction.
- We can concentrate on the development of problem-solving techniques. One way to define "stress" is "what people experience when they are called on to solve a problem." When you improve problem-solving skills, you have automatically given people improved stress management tools.
- We can concentrate on resistance. Those with limited training may provide great ideas for stress reduction that people never implement. Therapists understand that resistance is part of the change process and therefore can factor it into the training program.
- Our programs leave room for the development of individualized strategies. Unlike those who offer canned programs, therapists have the necessary knowledge to provide participants a range of approaches and then help them come up with their own tailor-made strategies.
- Our workshops can include experiential exercises, not just cognitive experiences, because, as therapists, we are not afraid of affect.
- Finally, we can attend to the change process in general. The therapist's expertise is helping people change, which involves not only resistance but also helping people develop workable strategies that will actually lead to long-term behavior changes.

We offer three separate packages. The first is brief, perhaps a half-day. It offers a primarily cognitive experience. Its advantage to the company is that it requires little time and money. The advantage to us is that, as an entry-level service, it may lead to more work with the company after its employees have an opportunity to become more familiar with us.

The second package covers the same material but involves enough time to accomplish the individual goals mentioned. This workshop could last a day or longer, depending on what is negotiated with the company and/or team taking the seminar.

The third package could last a number of days, again depending on the participants and their goals. It is designed for a management team and is intended not only to teach about stress management but also to be an intervention in problems specific to the team. During the first day, the program is a lot like package 2. Attention is paid to stress, its potential toxicity, and to individual stress management needs. However, it also can serve as a shared experience for the team. Then, on subsequent days, the team can focus on solving the team's own unique problems.

The consultant's role during those subsequent days is to facilitate group interactions during the meeting and to help team members use the problem-solving techniques learned during the formal toxic stress management training. This experience can serve to integrate the team's new learning into their actual behavioral repertoire. It also can serve as an enhancement to team functioning.

Trauma Response Teams

Traumas happen everywhere, including at work. People have serious accidents, workers assault each other, a coworker commits suicide, banks are held up, a dismissed worker occasionally returns to work with a gun in hand, and so on. Employees exposed to trauma suffer at the time. Worse, they are vulnerable to developing a posttraumatic stress disorder (PTSD). We know that most people seen within 24 to 48 hours of a trauma can be led through relatively simple procedures that drastically lower the risk of PTSD. What people need will depend on the nature of the experience, their emotional and physical proximity to the trauma, and the personal meaning of the trauma to them.

That 24- to 48-hour posttrauma period of high emotional distress is not the time when companies should do their planning for how to respond to trauma. Planning must take place beforehand, when heads are clear. This planning can begin by having a therapist educate the company's leaders about the advantages of having such a plan. The therapist can talk about the nature of trauma and about how PTSD develops. He or she can outline the long-term debilitating effects of trauma on employee performance and employee retention. Many employees quit their jobs after a trauma, not wanting to revisit the trauma site and experience its effect on their anxiety level. Whenever this happens, the employer must bear a significant expense in replacing them. Having a trauma response plan in place can help vulnerable employees and simultaneously protect the employer from large, unnecessary expenditures. It is a win–win situation that costs the employer little more than a day's consultation and training to put into place.

The next step is planning to set up a trauma response team: a group of company employees entrusted to anticipate and respond to possible traumas. The team is responsible for evaluating specific situations to determine if any action should be taken and, if so, what action to take. It sets up ways to evaluate employees for various levels of intervention, which range from simple informing, to enhanced critical incident debriefing, to referral for individual professional services.

Finally, the team is responsible for sharing information with the public when appropriate. How this is handled may have an immense impact on how the company is perceived by the public for years to come. Johnson & Johnson's response to the Tylenol poisoning episodes several years ago was a classic example of coolness under fire. Their straightforward and open response to the problem was not only the right thing to do but may well have saved the Tylenol product line. Having a trauma response plan in place increases the likelihood of having a cool enough head to communicate appropriately with the public in an emergency.

The bank president had seen the effects of armed holdups on employees before. When this one happened, he took action immediately. He arranged for me to meet with the branch team present at the robbery. I saw them the next evening and again a few days later for follow-up, using an enhanced critical incident debriefing procedure.

After brief introductions and a discussion of the purpose of our meeting, I asked each member of the group to tell the story of the robbery. It was interesting to watch the group piece the events together. No one individual had all the information. Just getting all the pieces in place seemed to help people feel better.

Then we did another go-round. This time we discussed feelings—the feelings during the robbery and the feelings since. Sharing these feelings with each other provided a level of understanding that was not available from their other sources of support. Again, one could see a growing sense of mastery over the experience.

As a natural outgrowth of examining their feelings, participants discussed the "crazy" symptoms that were plaguing them. They talked of trouble sleeping, nightmares, crying, and irritability. One woman who lived alone talked of becoming "paranoid" and of not answering the phone when it rang. All reported residual anxiety as well as anxiety over the meaning of their symptoms. When they learned that all of these were normal reactions to trauma—to the experience of having the myth of safety rudely ripped away—the expressed sense of relief in the room was palpable. Their education on this subject came partly from me and partly from one another. This new information did not make the symptoms instantly disappear. But now at least they did not have the added problem of worrying about being "crazy."

We looked at their sources of emotional support. All had important people in their lives, but each reported some disappointment with their loved ones' efforts to be supportive. Loved ones tended to want to shush them. My role at that point was to help them understand the anxiety people experience in response to *other people's* trauma. People do not want to recognize that tragedy really *can* happen to *anyone*—that the myth of safety *really is a myth*. That reluctance to admit vulnerability leads many loved ones to behave insensitively. This information helped the group stop taking the behavior personally. Then we talked about how they could let significant others know what they needed.

Next, we turned our attention to dealing with the anxiety of going back to work. Some form of desensitization was necessary. Because I like to do hypnotherapy, that was the approach we used. Other methods could work just as well. Whereas the bank branch had become associated with the terror of the robbery, the trance work helped the participants remember the calm and confidence that were more often a part of their experience in that setting.

Finally, we dealt with empowerment. One of the problems for those who go through trauma is a sense of helplessness. Action plans help to overcome helplessness. A problem relating to the trauma is identified, and those involved develop and carry out a plan to solve that problem. The problem does not have to be huge. It is the successful carrying out of an action plan, rather than passive submission in the aftermath of terror, that empowers people.

One of the problems these workers reported was the insensitivity of some bank executives (not the president!) to their feelings immediately after the robbery. We created a plan by which they could safely give these individuals some feedback.

The outcome was that people were able to go back to work. They were reasonably comfortable and the bank was able to retain experienced, talented employees.

Health Promotion Programs

Ken Pelletier, a professor of psychology at Stanford, has done a great deal of work with corporate America on developing programs in the workplace that promote healthy practices among employees. His consulting clients have included some of the largest companies in America. His programs focus on such things as smoking cessation, coronary heart disease risk reduction, exercise programs, and the like. In *Mind as Healer; Mind as Slayer* (1992), in particular, Pellitier's work in stress management is seminal. His review of 47 workplace health promotion programs (Pellitier,

1991) shows overwhelming evidence of the money-saving aspects of these programs for employers as employees benefit from improved health.

At his 1993 workshop, "Practical Strategies for Health Promotion," Pelletier talked about the role that therapists can play in such programs. He noted that our expertise in behavior change was a key element in making such programs successful. He also discussed the need to appreciate organizational aspects of the endeavor and yet clearly showed that a Ph.D. in organizational dynamics is not necessary to make such programs work. Pelletier's success is strong testimony to the capacity of those who understand behavior change to make a significant contribution in this area.

Peak Performance Consultation

Executives and sales personnel sometimes face situations that demand bursts of high performance. What one person regards as a high-performance challenge may not be challenging to someone else. It is the perspective of the doer that matters. For some it might be a special presentation. For CEOs it might be an especially difficult meeting with the Board of Directors. There are a wide variety of possibilities. We can help people get ready in many ways.

My favorite approach to such problems is to use hypnotherapy, both personally and with my clients. My own experience speaks to its efficacy. These days, I speak in public frequently and enjoy doing so. However, the first time I was asked to speak in public, four months after taking my first job as a psychologist, I was terrified. It was a simple PTA talk, the kind that, by now, I have given a hundred or more times. That first time, though, it filled my entire Christmas holidays with dread.

Today, my comfort level is much higher, and yet that anxiety (though not the dread) still exists, especially for difficult presentations. Prior to one major (at least it was to me) presentation in 1984, I obtained a consultation in peak performance for myself. I was taught how to take myself into trance to take control of my performance. This work involved achieving a sense of peacefulness, picturing past successes, and then rehearsing successful images for the upcoming presentation. It continues to be a part of my routine today.

Performance consultation is a powerful service we can offer to executives and others who must occasionally operate at their peak. We can help them prepare for those challenging experiences in a variety of ways. Hypnotherapy is one. You might use other approaches, such as deep muscle relaxation and imagery, or cognitive behavior modification (relative to thoughts of failure). There are many possibilities.

Process Consulting

Process consulting cuts across many of the kinds of services we can provide to business. During the VACP Marketing Project, Tom DeMaio, Ph.D., then president of VACP, did an outstanding 4-hour training program for our volunteers on process consulting that opened about 35 sets of eyes to the possibilities that might await them in the field of business consulting.

Tom noted that most consultation is seen as experts giving sage advice. It is quite content-oriented. Our expertise is not business content, *nor does it have to be.* Business already has lots of experts in business. Our fundamental expertise is in the *process in human interactions,* noticing how things go rather than what goes. Looking at the world through that particular prism shows us much important information that others often miss. We can help them to see it.

Process consulting is usually not something that is asked for. If employers knew about and understood process consultation, perhaps they would ask for it. But they usually don't. Instead, the initial request is likely to be for training, which the company hopes will be the solution to the problem as the company has defined it. When they ask for training, it gives you the chance to say something like "Tell me more about the problem." Off you go.

Listen carefully to the problem. People love to be listened to. This is a key way to gain entry into a company. As you listen, listen beyond the words to hear the problem. Do not just accept the description at face value, any more than you would sitting in your therapy office. You have done this kind of listening before. As you listen, you will begin to formulate a description in your own mind of what the real problem is. You will consider such issues as: how power is handled in the company, what the leadership styles are, how conflict is dealt with, what forms of communication are sanctioned, what the level of company-wide morale is, how the organization approaches problem solving, how the company is structured, and what personnel issues may exist.

Your understanding of the problem will lead you to decide how to respond. However, in process consulting, as in therapy, the keys are to engage the client(s) in the process of problem solving, help them to understand what is happening, and guide them in the selection of ways *they,* not you, can solve the problems. Sound familiar?

Self-Esteem Development

There is a consultant in Cincinnati who works with employees in groups on the subject of improving self-esteem. He is not a trained professional.

In fact, he took the business over from his father. He gets $5,000 a day for seminars. While this may not be a realistic starting fee for you, it gives you an idea how such services can be valued by business.

Communication

Many companies work extremely hard on their communication skills, developing the best doggone set of employee publications possible. These companies fail to understand genuine communication. While they focus on top-down message sending, we know that true communication is a feedback loop. We know how much more likely it is for our message to be received after we have listened. As Steven Covey (1989) writes: "Seek first to understand, then to be understood." Communication is our stock-in-trade. Skills that we take for granted are often sorely lacking in the business community. Imagine the increase in productivity that better communication could generate.

Coaching Interpersonal Skills

As the VACP Marketing Study found, many supervisors earn their positions through technical competence rather than personal skills. Yet, personal skills are essential if supervisors are to win the support and cooperation of their people. We can help supervisors develop those skills, using a coaching format that calls on many skills honed in therapy training. In addition, we could develop a group consultation approach that might function much like the group supervision most of us experienced during graduate training. If you can help supervisors develop a mutually supportive system in which they actually consult one another about difficult situations, you will have performed a wonderful service for the company, the supervisors, and those being supervised.

Troubled Employees

Every employer has troubled employees. We can act as consultants to management about how to respond to these troubled employees. The difference between this service and a traditional EAP is that the focus is on helping the company respond to the employee rather than finding or providing services for the employee. For example, as noted earlier, in Chapter 5, David Wiggins, Ph.D., a therapist in the Manassas Group, helps adult ADHD individuals and their employers tailor the job to fit the employee's style.

Troubled Departments

Most companies have troubled departments. Because we are used to dealing with emotionally charged issues and know how to establish environments within which people can talk about emotionally difficult material, we are able to create and execute interventions that can solve group problems, especially when we think systemically.

Leaders in most businesses do not understand systems issues. Trapped in linear thinking, their response is often to hunt for a scapegoat (sound familiar?). We can help companies understand how to differentiate between problems that are organizationally or system-based and those that are genuinely in response to one individual.

Changing Corporate Culture

We are experts in change. We help people and families change all the time. Corporations often find that the way their company culture has evolved is now unsuitable in some key manner. The new orientation to corporate reengineering speaks to this question. (See, e.g., *Re-engineering the Corporation: A Manifesto for Business Revolution,* by Hammer and Champy [1993].)

Maybe there is too little trust, or not enough open dialogue. Maybe a business wants to shift from a management orientation to one of leadership. Maybe it wants to encourage more risk taking. We can help businesses know how to make needed changes. You may need additional training in this area, and that training is available. University Associates (see the Appendix) offers a workshop in "Facilitating Organizational Change" that I found extremely helpful. Creative Dimensions in Management (see the Appendix) offers a 2-day program that teaches how to use therapy skills in organizational change. My partner and two colleagues give this workshop rave reviews.

Insurance Adjusters in Disasters

An insurance company recently found out something that might seem obvious to us, were we to attend to it. Normally, in disasters, insurance adjusters rotate though the devastated area. This means that a claimant might deal with several adjusters during the course of settling a claim. Both claimants and adjusters find this to be upsetting *and* inefficient. When a company allowed one adjuster to follow the claim all the way through, establishing a trustable relationship with the claimant, they found that everybody benefited. The claimants were less upset. Adjusters were more efficient. The company saved money. Our role could be to bring this to the attention of other insurance companies and then sensitize adjusters to the psychological components of dealing with disaster victims.

Psychological Assessments for Executive Selection

As I mentioned in Chapter 9, Rodney Lowman, Ph.D., has offered a 1 day training program that most clinical psychologists would find sufficient to prepare them for this activity. He presents a conceptual framework and a methodology for individual assessments that help executives and companies to make good fits with each other. Many psychologists who consult to business find that this is a service that gets them in the door. Other opportunities follow.

CREATING YOUR OWN SERVICES: LOOKING FOR OPPORTUNITIES

Fifteen possible services within People-Consulting in the Workplace have been considered so far. My hope is that by reviewing these possibilities, you might begin to be able to envision yourself doing a few of them that fit your talents and interests. The list offered only scratches the surface. You are limited only by your own imagination. Let me show you a method to feed your imagination further.

Recall our friend the newspaper. Many opportunities are announced daily in the headlines, if you learn how to recognize them. Remember that the newspaper is basically a journal that reports human problems. The business section of newspapers reports on problems that people in business care about. Let's look at some examples of headlines.

Working Women Feel Cheated

This story in my local paper came from a wire service. It outlined how women experience considerable stress in response to unfair pay, lack of recognition, limited training opportunities, child care issues, and the "glass ceiling" that exists in many companies. This story presents us with at least two business opportunities.

The first might be to devise an intervention about attitudes toward women within particular companies. Such a program would help companies see how talent already present within their employees is currently being wasted as a result of unnecessary psychological barriers called prejudices. An effective program would need to go well beyond speeches and deal with issues relating to attitude change that are our bread and butter.

One model of culture change that some therapists are using goes somewhat as follows. For whatever reason, a company has made the decision to make a culture change. Deciding to and knowing how to are quite different. Some companies bring in a team of therapists to work with the top executives, using many traditional therapy techniques to help the executives change attitudes from the old culture to the new. While the goal is to make a change in the work environment, these therapists and executives will examine any aspect of the executives' lives that might interfere with the goal.

A second business opportunity that this headline and news story represent is a seminar or other training format for professional women on self-empowerment. The participants would come from different companies. You could help them process their experiences and look for ways to turn disadvantages to their advantage. To prepare for this work, you might interview women who have been successful to see what they can tell you about the process of overcoming prejudice based on one's gender.

All Work and No Play? Not on Office Computers

This article tells about a problem some companies have when large numbers of employees do their work on personal computers. It seems that sometimes employees spend a significant part of their workday playing computer games. Some have even purchased a program that will throw a spreadsheet up on the screen at the push of a button, in case the boss should suddenly appear. Of course, the spreadsheet is completely bogus.

These employees are behaving like children. The article reported that bosses tend to react to them as if they were children, sneaking around to catch employees playing. A game of cops and robbers has been put in play. Without recognizing it, supervisors have allowed immature behavior by employees to set the emotional/behavioral tone of the office.

A therapist who understands systems theory can readily see how this set of interactions developed and help the supervisor generate a better response. Such a therapist would encourage an adult response by the supervisor to employees' childish behavior. In this case, such a response would go something like: "John, I know that you are spending work time on computer games. Help me understand that." Or, if it is a group issue, the supervisor could call a meeting and say something like: "We all know that many individuals in this room are spending time playing games on their computers. This meeting is not about getting people in trouble. It's about solving a problem. The law of nature in business is that, for the company and all of our jobs to survive, our company must use its resources wisely. Playing games on company time doesn't seem like a wise use of resources. How can we solve this problem?" The ridiculousness of playing on company time will become instantly apparent when the issue is approached in an adult manner. When it is approached out of an attitude of anger and retribution, employees will only become defensive.

Someone who understands psychological issues can more easily spot the real issues in this kind of problem and offer guidance to the employer. Imagine the improvements in productivity and psychological well-being that can grow out of this simple intervention. The supervisor, perhaps caught up in the emotion of the transaction, will be able to stand back and gain perspective. Employees do not really feel self-respect when they are spending company time playing games. They feel their best when spending work time doing good work. The supervisor, also a human being, will be less frustrated and more in control of his or her own behavior. Finally, this intervention might serve to identify underlying issues within the department or company that may have inadvertently encouraged immature behavior.

Latest Addition to Executive Suite
Is Psychologist's Couch

This headline appeared in the August 29, 1994, *Wall Street Journal*. The story reported about an industrial psychologist by the name of Dr. Bradford Smart. He apparently has established a thriving practice doing personal coaching of top executives of major corporations. For his services, he was reported to earn between $3,000 and $6,000 per day.

The people Dr. Smart coaches are talented executives having interpersonal difficulties with colleagues and others such that performance becomes a problem. His approach seems quite sensible. First, he does 360 degree feedback. This means that he and the executive seek behavioral feedback from superiors, colleagues, those who report to the executive, and, when appropriate, customers or clients. He also has them take objective psychological tests. He and the executive review all the data and set goals. He then coaches the executive through making the desired changes, using, I suspect, traditional therapeutic methods. Which part of this program could you not do?

Of course, remember that the company is the client. The executive must know this. Honest agreements about the limits of confidentiality need to be made. However, it helps to know that usually a company does not care about the intimate details of the executive's life. The company cares about results—whether or not changes needed by the company are being made. You need to discuss rules about boundaries with both the company and the executive before accepting the consultation. If management gets too nosey and does not respond to the established boundaries, walk away from that company. It will be nothing but trouble.

Because there are overlapping interests between the executive and the company, executive coaching is usually a viable project. If the executive discovers that the changes the company wants are personally undesirable or impossible, you have helped that executive discover, in a constructive way, a piece of reality that more often is discovered in painful ways. Without you, the usual "plan" is for the executive to "screw up" one too many times and get fired. Here, if the changes are not desirable or feasible, a change in employment can be made in a planful, constructive way.

In addition, you as consultant must be comfortable with the value system of the company. This means that you have to make some decisions about what values make sense in the workplace versus, say, the family. Remember that employers play a different role in the worker's life than his family does. Work is not intended to be a place where people are loved and accepted for who they are. Employees must execute their duties competently. When they do not, everyone else in the company is hurt.

If, on the other hand, the company's value is to drive people until they drop, you may not want to participate. However, before you walk away, you might want to take a shot at helping the company recognize the problems they are creating for themselves with that value. Some companies may be responsive to an intervention around that issue and others may not. Do not do the coaching if you, the company, and the executive cannot settle upon a mutually acceptable value system.

CEO Counselor Sees Field Change with the Times

This story, in our local paper, related the career of Mortimer Feinberg, who has been an industrial psychologist since 1950 and has worked with the leaders of some of America's largest companies (Rosenberg, 1995). Listening appears to have been the cornerstone of his career. The article noted: "Clients bring a variety of problems to his office: disagreements with superiors or subordinates, marital difficulties, even problems with mistresses" (p. F4). The CEO of one firm who used his services called him a healer, a confidant, totally trustworthy. "As a result of using him, we have had enormous success in attracting, retaining and keeping some of the best management we could possibly have . . . " (p. F4). What more needs to be said?

People Work Differently Overseas and You Have to Know How

This article, in our local paper's business section, highlights some issues therapists may take for granted but that business people may not recognize. People behave differently in different cultures. A behavior in one culture may have different meaning in another. Many Americans have failed to appreciate cultural differences and have unknowingly or unintentionally insulted foreign hosts in a variety of ways. Imagine the consequences such behavior can have in doing business.

Perhaps you have lived overseas or traveled extensively or emigrated here from another country. Those experiences can be put to use in sensitizing Americans sent overseas by their companies, an increasingly frequent experience. You could also work with their families, since a great many executives come home early from assignments because family members could not handle the stresses involved in the foreign culture.

Your task would be to help employees bound for overseas duty to recognize that cultural differences exist. Different cultures, for example, have different rules about physical space. People in some cultures stand very close to each other while talking while people in other cultures stand much farther apart. The tacit rules that govern how people may touch each other vary from culture to culture. Some people never think about these things. Then their behavior is misinterpreted as intentionally insulting instead of simply ignorant.

SUMMARY

In this chapter we have identified some of the services you could provide to business. We have also looked at how those services actually link up with expertise that you already have. I hope that this sampling of possibilities (among countless others) has increased your interest in People-Consulting. As you work through the next two chapters, you will develop ways to overcome many of the barriers standing between you and successful service delivery to the business world. In my experience, overcoming barriers has significantly enhanced my enthusiasm.

Chapter 11

Making a Business Plan for People-Consulting in the Workplace

In Chapter 7 we developed a business plan for delivering traditional services to your community. You will also need a business plan for the part of your practice devoted to People-Consulting in the Workplace. Once more, we will use the structure of the business plan (see Box 11.6 on pages 251–254) to discuss many of the issues you need to consider. Because some of the issues are different, the business plan form offered at the end of this chapter is a bit different from the one used in Chapter 7.

WHAT BUSINESS ARE YOU IN?

Step 1 is to figure out what kinds of services you want to provide within the general area of People-Consulting in the Workplace. You will see in the next chapter that you do not want this list to be too rigid, or else it may prevent you from responding to the needs of individual companies. However, you do need to have a reasonably well-developed sense of the kinds of services you want to provide. Doing so helps you to establish a sense of identity with flexible boundaries.

The same three fundamental principles apply in identifying services here as applied in Chapter 7:

- Learn what issues are of urgent concern to potential client companies.

- Have a clear idea of the benefit or value your service has for a business. They buy on the basis of value, just as individuals do.
- Make it easy for a company to begin a relationship with you by including at least some entry-level services in your mix.

How do you research the market? By reading Chapter 10, you have already begun. The list of services presented in Chapter 10 is based on my research for this book and research that my partner and I did in developing Peak Performance Consultation. Having no guide to follow, my partner and I spent 18 months planning Peak Performance Consultation. Much of our early time was spent conceptualizing the general field, as reviewed in Chapter 9, and then figuring out what we could do that would have value. One of my goals in writing this book is to shorten your development time—dramatically.

In developing our People-Consulting services, Lou and I examined our training and previous episodic experiences in business consulting, talked with other clinicians who had made the transition, read in a variety of areas, took additional training, considered our experiences with the Virginia Marketing Project, read the newspaper for daily business opportunities, and talked with people in the business community to get their reactions and thoughts. We used this information in a long series of discussions between us. Each of these methods can work for you, as well.

Over the next few weeks, then, read the newspaper with an eye for ideas. Read some business oriented books, such as *The Healthy Company* by Bob Rosen (1991) and *The Paradox of Success* by John O'Neil (1993). Talk with some colleagues and seek out a business person or two, mainly to "pick their brain."

If you think you don't know any business people, think again. Do you have neighbors? Friends? Relatives? Do you coach Little League? Belong to your child's PTA? Do you shop in any retail establishments? Who sold you your house? Surely, all the people you know are not therapists! What do those other people do for a living? Begin to make a list. Call a few people you feel comfortable with. Say something like: "Hi. This is Sally. I'm thinking about expanding my services, and I need to bounce some ideas off somebody who knows about the business world. Could I take you to lunch?" Remember, the goal of this conversation is *not* to get them to buy your services. It is to get their advice. Most people are flattered to have their opinions honestly sought.

The real estate agent my wife and I found to help us buy our home and who helped me find office space as well has become a friend. She is married to the CEO of a local company with about 200 employees. He agreed to have lunch with Lou and me and provided responses to our ideas from the perspective of a well-seasoned businessman.

Hearing how he deals with some of the people issues that come up in his company was an invaluable experience. We also heard about some of his experiences with training consultants. He helped us realize that our plan to hire a salesperson (so that we could avoid the anxiety of the sales process) was doomed to failure. "To sell *these* services, you must sell yourself." he said. Unfortunately, that made sense. Still, I responded: "But I'm not a sales guy!" His answer to that was: "What do you mean? You've been selling me for the last hour!" That comment alone was worth the price of the lunch.

As with your traditional service plan, one part of defining your business is determining what services you will *not* provide. No matter how flexibly you might listen to a company's needs, you will hear some requests that do not fit who you are. For example, we were once approached by a large local company that was looking for training for their employees. The Vice President for Human Resources was the decision maker, and he liked us. However, the content of the training that was needed was technical and classroom-oriented. While we are a training company, we did not want to be *that* kind of training company. We could have taken the contract and then looked for vendors, but we turned it down.

Besides the fact that the task was too far outside our core business, the contract was too big. *Too big?* Yes. Had we responded to the request, all of our eggs would have been in that one basket. We would have been too dependent upon that one company, because the demands for service, even if we got vendors to help us, would have consumed most of our time. The business we have defined for ourselves is designed to have several concurrent clients. This approach provides us financial protection from the potential disaster of losing our only major customer. For your own reasons, you may define your business differently. However, as you define your services, you will want to consider their scope.

As mentioned earlier, a psychologist I know in New York focuses only on Trauma Response Plans for companies in her geographical area. She helps the companies establish the plans and then provides additional services if traumas actually occur. She has found that she can fill 30%–40% of her time doing that work, spending the balance of her week doing therapy. She does not accept requests to provide other services. For her, Trauma Response Plans are the goal. For Peak Performance Consultation, such plans represent an entry-level service, one way of establishing a relationship we hope will lead to other business. This different emphasis is based on having a different definition of our business, which was based on our own needs and preferences. This whole discussion illustrates how defining your services helps you make decisions.

Now let yourself do some brainstorming. Better yet, find a buddy and brainstorm together. If you are extremely lucky, you will have a partner as talented and emotionally supportive as I do. If not, network. Find a colleague who may also be interested in People-Consulting in the Workplace. You do not have to go into business together in order to go through some of the conceptualization process together. Having that extra brain to work with will lead to better ideas for both of you than either would develop alone. If you find you are a good fit for the business community, what would stop you from becoming partners just for this component of your practice?

If you do not go into partnership, you may worry that you will be generating competition. Hope that you do, for at least two reasons. First, we discussed earlier how competition breeds business by normalizing the process. The more companies that use People-Consulting in the Workplace style services, the greater the demand will become. As I said, I look to the day that it becomes as normal for businesses to have psychologically oriented consultation as it is to have financial consultation.

Second, you and your friend may refer to each other. Sometimes this will be because your friend does something you do not. Or there may be reasons your friend cannot provide the service and refers to you. Recently, a colleague I met through the Virginia Marketing Project had a CEO for a therapy client who was beginning to want some help with his company. My colleague did not feel he could provide both services, so he gave the man my name. This may or may not lead to business for me, but the opportunity would not exist were it not for networking.

After doing some of the research suggested, use the same list-making method we used in Chapter 7. Make four lists: a list of your interests (see Box 11.1), a list of needs you have found in your community (see Box 11.2), a list of services you already know how to provide (see Box 11.3), and a list of services you already know are not for you (see Box 11.4). Look for items common to the first three lists as constituting your core list of services.

Remember that, as you develop your skills and specialties through additional training, mentoring, observation, and experience, you can add to the items on your list of services.

MISSION STATEMENT

Having conceptualized your services, you are now ready to begin considering a mission statement. What is the primary goal of your business, besides making a profit? What is its core reason for existing that will matter to potential clients? Remember that mission statements need to be brief. Brevity makes mission statements difficult to write because of the clarity

---

BOX 11.1. People-Consulting in the Workplace
Services That Command My Interest

1. _____
2. _____
3. _____
4. _____
5. _____
6. _____
7. _____
8. _____
9. _____
10. _____

---

of thought required. Do not get stymied by this task. It may take your unconscious several months to deliver, but, if you are patient and make occasional conscious efforts, it will.

Let me repeat the mission statement for Peak Performance Consultation first mentioned in Chapter 9: "We deal with the psychological barriers to productivity." We were very close to the initial offering of our

---

BOX 11.2. Results of Market Studies: Issues
of Urgent Concern to the Business Community

1. _____
2. _____
3. _____
4. _____
5. _____
6. _____
7. _____
8. _____
9. _____
10. _____

**BOX 11.3. People-Consulting in the Workplace:
Services I Know How to Do Now**

1. _____

2. _____

3. _____

4. _____

5. _____

6. _____

7. _____

8. _____

9. _____

10. _____

---

services before that statement came to us. At that point, our thinking crystallized in terms of what we are about. Now it seems easy.

IDENTIFYING AND ASSESSING YOUR COMPETITION

As with marketing traditional services, it is important to know who your competitors are and what relative strengths and weaknesses each of you has.

You face competition from four sources:

- Other external consultants like yourself
- Organizational development (OD) consultants
- National training companies with canned presentations
- Consultants internal to the company

Some external consultants will have training similar to yours, especially as this type of work becomes more popular among therapists. Other competitors will be individuals with training in OD. You will also run into consultants who have developed their skills within the business world and through life experiences. An excellent trainer with University Associates from whom I took a course on OD has a Ph.D. in English.

With regard to other consultants like you, one issue that will separate

---

BOX 11.4. People-Consulting in the Workplace: Services I Choose Not to Offer

1. _____
2. _____
3. _____
4. _____
5. _____
6. _____
7. _____
8. _____
9. _____
10. _____

---

you from them is timing. Many consultants get hired partly because they happen to show up at the right time. Doing your homework in terms of reading about business issues and local companies may improve your timing. If a company is making noises about downsizing, you may want to go talk with the company leaders. If a company is getting ready for a strike and you happen to know a key player, it might be a good time to make a call. If there is an acquisition being made in your area, you might want to explore their interest in programs designed to help employees of the purchased company adapt to the new corporate culture.

If two or more of you show up at the right time, another determining factor is the relationship that develops between you and the decision maker. Good listening and practical, effective solutions build good relationships.

Do not underestimate the skills and psychological knowledge some of your nontherapist competitors have who have honed their skills via business and life experience. They may speak business lingo better than you do, and they sometimes have some good insights about people. We do not have a monopoly on insight. It is important to find ways to counter their skills and experience. Therefore, do not underestimate your own skills and experience. Many competitors, for example, will not have your depth of understanding of individual dynamics. This understanding of individual dynamics is critical to the success of business systems. Your extensive formal training in human change is a huge asset, as long as you can avoid the image of "shrink." In addition, you are likely to know more about how to facilitate emotionally based behavioral change. You may know more about providing personal feedback in constructive ways than many competitors. You won't always win the competition, but then you don't have to.

There are many consultants who know more about business than we do. We are not business experts in the same sense that they are. We are people experts. We bring something new to the table. By combining the business expertise of employers with our people expertise, we can make a new mix of skills and creativity that will result in big improvements in company performance.

Organizational development consultants' understanding of systems and groups may be superior to yours, depending upon what efforts you take to educate yourself in that area. Your understanding of individual issues may be superior to theirs. Determining which of you can better help to solve the problem may depend on the nature of the problem.

Most of us will be relatively inexperienced at business consulting (as compared to some of our competitors). While we do not need to parade it, we also do not want to hide the fact that we are in some ways new to this work. We need not and should not pretend to be something we are not. The key is to find a way to turn who we are to our advantage. Being willing to work harder is one time-honored way for new businesses to gain market share. Business people understand that new businesses are often willing to go the extra mile to earn a contract, and that can be appealing. They know you will take a special interest in their problems. Sometimes, you may want to offer a financial deal because you are new. One of our first Peak Performance projects was done at about half-price because we wanted that particular experience. The more established you become, the less necessary it is to offer significant discounts.

If you do decide to offer a discount, do not lead with it. Let the company raise the issue of expense, or you may raise an issue that did not concern them. Do not offer a discount in a manner that suggests you do not believe you are worth the original figure. That would suggest to the company that your service would be poor. They will never buy a service you believe to be shoddy, amateurish, or subpar. Offer the discount to earn market share for your new enterprise.

Some national training firms offer good programs. They come into town for a day, and for about $100/employee they can train a lot of people from several area companies. Employers have to make only a minimal investment in money and employee time. This is a good deal for companies that want just a handful of employees trained in something fairly straightforward. The downside is that these are *canned* programs. Everybody gets the homogenized version. If a company wants more than 20 employees trained, or if the problem requires more than simply training, the company might be better off to have you come on site.

Peak Performance custom-tailors everything we do for the particular company we are working with. We have found this to be a major selling point. You can see that both you and national training firms have advantages. Your task is to emphasize the value of the tailored approach, without knocking the alternative.

Finally, you may wonder why a company would hire you to consult if it has in-house OD consultants or an in-house EAP, some of which are beginning to widen their scope of service. There are a variety of reasons why you may get the nod.

Obviously, the in-house people have the advantages of cost and of already having a relationship with the company. Yet, sometimes a company prefers to use external resources because the nature of the project is particularly sensitive. Or it might be that the company feels the need for an external perspective. For example, most CEOs know that they are in danger of getting sanitized reports from people within the firm. They may want a perspective from an outsider who is not dependent on the CEO for his or her entire livelihood. Do not automatically disqualify yourself from working with companies with internal resources. You may be walking away from some nice contracts.

If you do connect with a company that has in-house staff, find a way to make them your allies. One strength you have in this regard is that you are not after a permanent relationship with their company. If you can find a way to leave the in-house staff empowered, your intervention will have a much higher likelihood of not getting sabotaged.

FINANCIAL POLICIES

Setting Your Fees

As with your traditional services, you will need to consider a number of factors in determining what to charge. Doing this in a competent manner can play a large role in determining whether your business is economically viable.

Costs

Review the list of expenses in Box 7.5. What *additional* costs might you have if you open a business consulting practice to supplement your therapy practice? You will have new marketing materials to prepare (see Box 11.5). You will probably want to have different stationery and business cards. They should look businesslike rather than "shrinky." They should not mention psychotherapy. You may want to get a logo created, which can be done for a few hundred dollars. (Call a graphic designer.) You may wish to put in a separate phone line. You may join some local business organizations such as the Chamber of Commerce or Rotary, which will require dues. You may join professional organizations, such as the Society of Psychologists in Marketing (SPIM). You may decide to take additional training. Review your malpractice insurance policy to see if it covers you when providing these services. If not, buy additional coverage. Some consultants buy "Errors and Omissions" coverage, which is a kind of malpractice policy. You may choose to upgrade your computer or hire additional office staff. And it may not hurt to buy a few business suits.

Your Income

How much business consulting do you want to do? Review your overall income goal. How much of your income do you want to derive from this part of your practice? How much time do you want to devote to it? As an example, my overall goal is to devote two days per week to business consultation. Since I figure I have 44 work weeks, I expect to devote 88 days to business consulting. Not all of that is likely to be billable time. However, what I do bill must cover a minimum of 40% of my income goal.

Competitors' Fees

Many clinicians I know essentially double their clinical rate. The rationale is that this charge covers the unreimbursed time that is inherent in do-

---

BOX 11.5. Possible Additional Expenses for People-Consulting in the Workplace

Marketing materials	$_____
New stationery	$_____
New business cards	$_____
Logo design	$_____
New phone line	$_____
Dues to business groups (e.g., Rotary, Chamber of Commerce)	$_____
Additional training	$_____
Additional insurance	$_____
New computer or other office equipment	$_____
Additional secretarial services	$_____
Unreimbursed time spent on sales calls and development of marketing materials	$_____
New clothes	$_____

ing People-Consulting in the Workplace. Unreimbursable time includes sales calls and much of the time involved in creating marketing materials and researching and developing programs. If you forget to build this time into your charges, you could easily wind up working at a loss compared to what you could earn selling your services in other ways.

By asking around, we learned that the minimum daily charge for our competitors with more business-oriented backgrounds is about $1,500 per day, which is also approximately double the clinical rate for many clinicians. However, I found that the *average* rate was more in the $2,000-per-day range, or about $225 per hour. This has become my target charge. Often I get it. Other times I am willing to negotiate downward to obtain a desired contract.

During our consultation with Saul Gellerman, we discussed fee structure. He declines to establish an hourly rate, telling potential clients: "Once I commit part of a day to you, I cannot use any part of the day for someone else." The rationale for this policy stems from the fact that he does business with large companies in different cities. A consultant who works locally has more flexibility in his or her schedule. You could consider developing a half-day rate if you did not like the idea of an hourly rate.

Also, recall some of the stories told earlier. Dr. Smart is charging between $3,000 and $6,000 per day, according to the *Wall Street Journal*. The self-esteem expert in Cincinnati is charging $5,000 per day for seminars. Another psychologist I know is also at the $5,000-per-day level for seminars to companies. In a conversation, not a sales call, with a vice president for a national company, I was told, "$2,000 a day is nothing if you can help solve a $10-million business problem. In fact, if you charge less than that, they may not take you seriously."

Don't forget that this book is being written in 1996, and the fees quoted are subject to becoming outdated. Fees may also be different depending upon the size of your city and the area of the country you live in. Therefore, do your own asking around. Talk with clinicians who have made the transition. When you do your exploratory talks with business people, ask them what rates they hear of being charged. As you take additional training, ask your trainers about their fees for consultation.

In establishing your charges, remember that, within reasonable limits, the issue is value, not cost. If the company can perceive your value — that what they invest in you will lead to a good return on that investment — you stand a good chance of getting what you ask for. For example, if they believe you can solve an expensive problem for less than they are losing by not solving it, they will probably spend the money. The return they are looking for will usually involve added value, and thus added productivity, within the workforce.

Negotiating a Fee

There is much more of a tradition of negotiating business consultation fees than therapy fees. Many therapists have little experience with negotiating and will need to develop some skills in that area. *Bargaining Games: A New Approach to Strategic Thinking in Negotiations* by Murnighan (1992) is an extremely helpful resource. Among other things, Murnighan points out that negotiations are not just about price. There are usually several factors involved, each of which can be a point of bargaining. For example, in negotiating a contract you will want to consider the following: who pays for training materials, who supplies training or work space, whether you are charging by contact hour (when you are actually with the client) or if you can charge for some or all preparation time, the kind of preconsultation assessment that is done, and so forth.

Murnighan, the Director of the Program on Conflict and Negotiation Research at the University of Illinois, also shares much useful information on the psychological components of negotiation and important ethical considerations. Finally, he supplies some fascinating exercises, some of which have found their way into my training programs.

One way to frame the negotiation about your fees is to ask the decision maker how much the problem is costing the company. By focusing attention on the cost of the problem, your fee looks smaller and more like an investment than an expense.

Payment Policies

Decide ahead of time how you want to handle collecting your fees. Sometimes it will make sense to bill by the project, especially if it is time-limited. For longer consultations, I bill monthly. Thus far, I have not had difficulties in collecting, though certainly that time will come. One way to minimize the occurrence of such problems is to negotiate the financial arrangement clearly up front. I usually put it in as part of my written proposal.

OFFICE POLICIES AND PROCEDURES

Your Image

Many business people have a biased view of members of our profession. They see us as strange or weird. If your behavior or image fits their expectation, do not expect to get many appointments. Sometimes people seem strange not because they *are* strange but because they come from a different culture. Therapists and business people have different cultures.

Since we are trying to enter the business culture, the onus is on us to learn their cultural norms. We can accommodate to these norms without losing our identity.

Your image will be communicated by how you talk, dress, and behave. It will also be communicated by your stationery, your marketing materials, the way you write, and how your phone is answered. For example, I changed the way my phone was answered from "Dr. Ackley's office" to "Dr. Ackley's office. Peak Performance Consultation." When I do written proposals, I write for a different audience than I do when writing for professional peers.

How do you learn about business culture norms? There are many ways. Lou and I hired a public relations expert to help us learn the ropes. I had hired her as a consultant to the Virginia Marketing Project and found her to be knowledgeable about business culture. She was of great help in preparing our marketing materials and stationery. Some of the specific materials she encouraged us to develop will be reviewed in the next chapter. We learned about the business culture from our conversations with people in the business world as we were getting started. Friends and relatives in the business world also provided good information. Reading books like *The Healthy Company, The Paradox of Success,* and *The Leadership Challenge* all widened my understanding (see the Appendix).

As you look for books on business to familiarize yourself with the issues, you may also want to peruse books available regarding business etiquette and dress. Consider, for example, *Your Executive Image: The Art of Self-Packaging for Men and Women* by Seitz (1992). With regard to dress, there is a change going on in the business world. Increasingly, companies are choosing to "dress down," or casually. Do not assume that is the case in any company you do not know well. Dress professionally for at least the first meeting. Also be aware that "dressing down" may mean different things to banks, investment firms, and law offices than to schools, stores, and government agencies.

Scheduling

If, like me, you choose to offer both traditional services and business consulting, scheduling can become difficult. The solution that I have developed rests on decisions about how I want to allocate my time. I am reducing my clinical work from 5 days per week to 2. Business consulting will be given 2 days per week, while activities relating to Building a Managed Care Free Practice seminars will be given 1 day per week.

Thus far, I have blocked off three mornings per week during which I do not accept clinical appointments. That time is used for writing, preparing seminars, making sales calls, preparing proposals, doing business presentations and consultations, and other varied activities. Sometimes consultations fall outside those slots. Many of them can be planned far enough in advance that they do not disrupt my clinical schedule.

Consider the issue of boundaries within your schedule. If I go out of town to do a seminar, which is usually on a Friday or Saturday, I block off compensatory time during the following week. If I did not, I would soon be overwhelmed. With good boundaries you are likely to succeed at juggling all the balls. Without them, things might get pretty confused.

BUSINESS ORGANIZATION

The same choices are available here as with traditional services. My partner and I have developed Peak Performance Consultation together, but we are not in business together in a legal sense. We share common expenses, such as stationery. However, we pay our own individual expenses and retain the fees we each generate. This arrangement gives us the advantage of combined resources and the freedom of individual decision making. It saves a lot of wasted energy in power struggles.

However, you may choose to operate entirely on your own, or within a larger, more formally organized group. It will depend upon your personality and your opportunities.

START-UP CAPITAL

We looked at the issue of capital in Chapter 7. The same issues apply. It is, shall we say, unlikely that companies will rush to your door the day you decide to do People-Consulting in the Workplace. As with all new businesses, money will go out for a while before it comes in. Figure out how much you need to get started. Include the costs of training, marketing materials, maybe a logo, any new equipment you decide to buy, new stationery and so forth. Figure in the uncompensated time that is a part of any new business (see Boxes 7.5 and 11.5).

Where will this money come from? During the long development time I went through, the income from my traditional practice sustained us, though, as indicated, at a declining level. As I mentioned before, I invested my unfilled clinical hours as well as a lot of "overtime" in planning my new ventures. This time was a resource I invested in my future. To what extent can your current income sustain you? What savings and credit resources do you have? Do not be afraid to use them.

(*continued from previous page*)

6. Pricing
   a. What are the costs of running your practice?
      (This information is in Box 11.5.) $_____
   b. What is your annual net income goal?   _____
      (If you set a goal, you have a chance to achieve it.)
   c. What is the range of your competitors' fees?   _____
   d. How many billable hours do you have available?   _____
   e. Given this information, what do you plan to charge per

   Day?   _____
   Half-day?   _____
   Hour?   _____

7. Factors that establish your identity with the business community (issues important for a therapy practice, such as parking and office location, are less important here because most of the time you will be going to the business, not them to you):

   a. New stationery? Yes _____ No _____
   b. How will your phone be answered? _____
   c. Do you need a new wardrobe? Yes _____ No _____
   d. Steps I will take to learn business culture norms:

   _____

   _____

   _____

   _____

8. Schedule
   a. Hours you will reserve for business consulting:

   _____

   b. Hours reserved for clinical work:

   _____

9. What kind of business structure will you use?

   _____ Solo practice _____ Partnership _____ Group practice
   _____ Institutional _____ Other (describe: _____

   _____)

(*cont.*)

(continued from previous page)

10. How will you fund your business? What resources do you have to call on (savings, credit cards, investment accounts, home equity accounts, etc.)?

    _____

    _____

    _____

    _____

    _____

    _____

11. What additional training would be helpful, either to your skills or your self-confidence?

    _____

    _____

    _____

    _____

    _____

    _____

Chapter 12

Marketing and Selling to Business

Many therapists who come to our seminars respond to People-Consulting in the Workplace in one of two ways: (1) "This is not for me" or (2) "This sounds great, but I have no idea how to get businesses to buy my services." Unfortunately, some therapists in the second category misplace themselves in the first just because they lack information on how to market and sell. They see what they believe to be an insurmountable barrier and immediately decide they are wrong for this diversification. This chapter is for them.

When I was hunting for office space to expand my private practice in 1980, landlords offered me rental figures in square footage charges. One space, for example, was offered at $6 per square foot (1980 dollars). To have a decent-sized office, a waiting room, and secretarial area, I wanted to have at least 700 square feet. Thinking that the square footage charges were *per month,* it appeared I faced rental charges of $4,200. "There is no way! How do those others do this?" I asked, about to give up. My friend in real estate told me that square footage is quoted as an annual figure, not a monthly one. That simple piece of information offered me great relief. My rent would only be $350 per month. Suddenly, having a practice was again feasible.

Similarly, the obstacles to connecting with business are smaller than *you* may imagine. A little information can make all the difference. We do not have to develop a level of expertise in marketing and selling comparable to professionals in these areas in order to have a viable business consulting practice.

CREATING A MARKETING PLAN

Remember that marketing is a two-step process of education. The first step involves learning the issues of urgent concern to potential clients. The second involves letting them know you have answers to their concerns. In Chapter 8 we looked at methods of marketing traditional services. Here we will apply the same principles to People-Consulting in the Workplace, taking you through the six questions of marketing that will guide you in developing your own marketing plan.

1. What Services Will You Provide?

Decisions about what services you will offer have been made as a part of creating your business plan. Having this list provides you with a focus for your work. It will help you answer the next five questions. When you get to the part of this chapter about selling, you will see why this list needs to be flexible in your mind, not a set of hard-and-fast limitations.

2. Who Are Your Potential Clients? What Is Your Market?

Decide who you want to sell your services to. That group of companies is your market. In order to define your market, you will need to consider several parameters, such as geographical reach, company size, and specific industries. In so doing, you will build a mental picture of your potential clientele. This picture can begin to replace the stereotypical picture many of us carry around of the "typical" business person.

What geographical area will you mainly serve? Will your market consist of local companies or will you travel? If you are willing to travel, *how far* are you willing to travel? Consider how the answer to this question will affect your life. Do you like traveling? Do you have a spouse and children? How is traveling likely to affect your family and marriage?

When we began planning for Peak Performance, I had fantasies of going all over a multistate region and perhaps all over the nation. My brother, Roger, who flies all over the world in his role as a sales manager for a national company, gave me good advice: "Dana, don't fly over a lot of business." This not only brought me down to earth, it saved a lot of time, money, and energy. So far, all the work I have done has been local, though we have made calls on two companies within an hour of Roanoke. Obviously, working in town makes it a lot easier, in terms of scheduling, to integrate People-Consulting in the Workplace with my clinical work.

In addition, I know people locally. That has implications for how

I choose to execute steps 5 and 6 of the marketing process. Saul Geller-
man has defined his market as national, and even international in scope.
He obviously has to factor travel time and expenses into his business plan.
As a result, his marketing approach, as you will see, is different as well.

What size companies will you serve? Again, my naive fantasies were
that we would be involved with your basic humongous company. This
has not proved to be true, which is good news given that there are a lot
more small companies than big ones. One of our first projects was with
a company of 18 people. They had the need and the money. Most of our
work has been with companies in the range of 200–300 employees. One
advantage of beginning with smaller companies is that it is easier to see
all parts of the system.

Gellerman, on the other hand, approached this decision differently.
He worked for IBM for a number of years. When he began his own consultation practice, it was natural for him to focus on big companies, who
became the majority of his clients.

Which industries will you work with? Some consultants specialize in
a particular industry. For example, they might be specialists in the banking industry or textiles. While I have not chosen that marketing strategy,
it is one to consider. Maybe there is an industry about which you already
have some content knowledge. As you gain experience in an industry, you
can establish yourself as an expert. You can make increasing numbers of
contacts within that industry, making it easier to obtain clients.

Whether you decide to go the "niche" market route may depend on
the opportunities in your area, whether there will be enough business to
sustain you, given your particular mix of business consulting/private therapy, and whether your comfort level lies in becoming really good at one
thing or enjoying a variety of experiences.

What services will you offer? How you define your market may relate to the services you offer. In determining your market, examine the
list of services you have selected to see in what directions they take you.
Trauma response plans, for example, may do better in high-risk industries than in companies in which the greatest danger is likely to be turning
on the computer. Process consulting, however, is applicable nearly
everywhere.

3. Where Can You Find Potential Clients?
Where Do They Hang Out?

If you want to communicate with potential clients, you need to be able
to find them. There are lots of ways to do this. First, check with your
local librarian about resource material that lists local employers, number
of employees, key executives, type of business, and so forth. Lists of major

employers are often found in local newspapers, local business journals, and sometimes local magazines. Your local Chamber of Commerce may be willing to give you its list of members. However, you may have to join to get it. This is not a bad idea because many business people attend Chamber meetings.

There are a number of other organizations designed for business people—Rotary International, Kiwanis, management associations, and the Jaycees are examples. Toastmasters International gives you a chance to gain speaking skills and form relationships at the same time. Local health care coalitions might be worth your consideration. These are organizations of businesses alarmed by galloping health care costs, who work together to find ways to respond to the problem.

Another place business people "hang out" is the business section in your local paper. Your area may also have a business journal. For example, in our area the *Blue Ridge Journal* is written strictly for a business audience.

You can also find business people in their offices and factories. Even if there were no ethical question, we still would not consider showing up at private homes to talk to people about coming in for therapy—because it is not cost-effective. However, businesses expect vendors to show up to talk to them about possible services. It is cost-effective for us to do so because of the large concentration of possible business in one place and the attractive financial payoff in landing an account. In the section of this chapter on selling, we will look at how to get an appointment and what to do when you get there.

Another place business people might hang out is at events you create. Our local Chamber of Commerce cosponsors workshops with eager vendors-to-be who want an opportunity to demonstrate their services. The vendor bears the expense but has the backing of the Chamber so that members can assume the program has some merit.

Potential clients hang out with vendors with whom they already do business. An EAP has their office in our building because they want proximity to the Manassas Group. They have introduced us to one potential client who was dealing with a troubled department within his 1,600-employee company. It was a problem the EAP could not help them with. However, if we are successful, that helps the EAP's relationship with the client company.

Banks are another vendor that businesses are likely to use. I have been involved as a customer in the private banking program of one bank for years. In one of their newsletters, they ran an article on the financial steps that aging CEOs of family businesses should take as leadership-succession issues begin to arise. A bell went off in my head. A classic business/family therapy problem is that families who own businesses get riled up and agitated as succession issues develop. The CEO often avoids succession planning because it forces simultaneous consideration of issues related to death. Entrepreneurs, who have devoted their lives to creating and building, may find it even more challenging to consider death than others do. The adult children, who usually have been thinking that they could "do it better" for years, want Dad or Mom to let go sooner. This struggle for control and empowerment, a normal family process, is intensified in family businesses. Imagine that you are like Prince Charles—in your late 40s and still a prince, not the king. I talked with my private banker, who confirmed that too often family business people do not take the financial steps they should, apparently for psychological reasons. The bank and I are now exploring ways to partner our services for such individuals.

4. What Value Does Your Service Have for Potential Clients?

Inherent in the descriptions of services in Chapter 10 is the value that your services can have to the company. This value will not be primarily in the human good you can do, although you are likely to hear talk in that direction. Do not fall for it. It is highly unlikely you will ever make a sale solely on doing human good. You will make sales because your services lead to increased profit. This has little to do with morality. It has to do with the reasons that businesses exist. They exist to make a profit. Were it not for profit, businesses would not exist and people would not have jobs. Goods and services would not be available. Fortunately, doing good for the people in the company by increasing psychological skills of leaders and staff often leads to increased profits.

> During one sales call, a human resources executive phrased the question this way: "What is the value-added to my company of your providing this service?" He wanted to know how his company would be better as a result of my intervention, a reasonable question. His company had been purchased by a larger one. Employees were experiencing great stress adjusting to the new company's culture. I offered to help the company design a program that would help employees to let go of their emotional ties to the old culture. The value-added was that employee productivity would be improved once employees broke through the barrier of grieving for the old culture.

How will your services lead to higher profits? Basically, you will help remove psychological and interpersonal barriers to productivity and creativity. Bad things—such as absenteeism, poor morale, passive-aggressive behavior, violence, and sabotage—will decline. Good things—

such as communication, commitment, enthusiasm, respect, customer service, and keeping the good employees—will increase.

All this is true. If you do not believe it, read *The Healthy Company* (see the Appendix). Once we believe it, all we have to do is to figure out how to tell potential clients.

5. How Can You Communicate About the Value of Your Service?

Lou and I started finding an answer to this question by consulting the public relations professional I had hired to help VACP with the Virginia Marketing Project. She taught us some getting started steps: "You need a leave-behind." "What's that?" we asked. "It's what you leave behind after a sales call so they don't forget you were there," she replied. That made sense.

"What should be in it?" we wondered. "You need (1) a list of services, (2) a fact sheet describing Peak Performance Consultation, and (3) a biographical sketch for each of you. In addition, descriptions of each major service would be good. All this should be in an attractive folder that is bigger than 8½ × 11 so it doesn't get lost on your prospect's desk. Finally, you need to get a logo, preferably professionally designed, to put on the folder and your stationery."

We took her advice. We assembled each of the pieces she suggested and got her feedback on them. In the pages that follow, I have reproduced these pieces. While you are unlikely to do yours just like ours, at least you will not have to reinvent the wheel.

List of Services

In crafting the language for our list of services (see Figure 12.1), the goal was to give potential clients a vision of how we could be helpful. We also wanted to normalize the use of our services rather than feed the notion that pathology was the issue. Rather than focus only on bad things that happen, we wanted to build a vision of additional good things that could happen. This approach would help us appeal to companies that are constantly striving for improvement as well as companies in pain.

We have grouped our services into three sets to help potential clients see a breadth of offerings. If their initial interest relates to individual skill issues (training), they can find something of interest. If instead they are ready for attention to be paid to systemic issues, they can find items there as well. The set of "Consultations" provides potential clients with another way to visualize using our services.

There is a mix of entry-level services and longer-range possibilities.

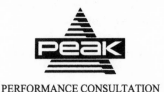

Dana C. Ackley, Ph.D.
(540) 774-1927

Louis A. Perrott, Ph.D.
(540) 989-8896

PERFORMANCE CONSULTATION

SERVICES OFFERED

Peak Performance Consultation helps companies develop their skills in creating work environments that summon the best from their people. We focus on the development of both company and individual strengths. In so doing we offer the following services:

Individual Skill Development Seminars:

    Conflict Management
    Toxic Stress Syndrome
    Transforming from Manager to Leader
    Becoming a Communicator: A Two-fold Process

Corporate Skill Development:

    Creating a Trauma/Crisis Corporate Response Plan
    How to Downsize without Losing Your Shirt
    Diagnosing Organizational Flaws (and fixing them)
    Changing Corporate Culture

Consultations:

    Mutual Adaptation for Results
    Peak Performance Training
    Coaching Interpersonal Skills
    Troubled Employees

3635 Manassas Drive, Suite A • Roanoke, Virginia 24018 • FAX (540) 989-8893

FIGURE 12.1. List of services for Peak Performance Consultation.

Some companies may have used consultants like us before. If so, they may be ready psychologically for a more extensive intervention than a company for whom this is all new.

If items on the list of services offered are unclear to you, refer back to Chapter 10. Each item is discussed there, with the exception of Mutual Adaptation for Results. Mutual Adaptation for Results is designed to introduce the concept that companies do best when they realize that it is not just employees who must adapt to the company. Companies must also adapt themselves to the skills, talents, and temperaments of the people they hire. This is a systemic concept.

Fact Sheet

A fact sheet is designed to present your consultation company. It needs to be brief! Limit yourself to one page and, even at that, include lots of white space. If it looks like a lot of work to read, many people won't make the effort. While the fact sheet has different parts, each part speaks to the *benefits* potential candidates can expect from using your services. *People buy on the basis of benefits.* This is not a place to emphasize methods. You will discuss methods in person, during a sales call, after significant interest has been established.

Our Fact Sheet (see Figure 12.2) begins with our mission statement (slightly reworded). To help make the statement's meaning clear, we expand it by speaking to both the systemic and individual skill levels. The language we use is designed to help readers visualize an exciting outcome in using our services.

The next section normalizes the need for our services. The last thing we want to do is suggest that only "sick" companies need us. Not only would that arouse the shame barriers we are working so hard to lower, but it would be untrue. All companies struggle with the issues outlined in that paragraph. We want them to see how using our services will provide solutions that have not previously been available to them.

Next, we work to differentiate ourselves from our competition. We do so by emphasizing the strengths we bring to the table. The discussion of our strengths provides an outline of our approach to doing business: we are experts in change who develop individualized programs based on solid assessments of what the problem really is. This section again concludes with a comment on benefits.

Finally, we give a brief description of who we are. Since our background and credentials will be detailed in the biographical sketch, here the discussion can be brief. If our company had a longer history, we would describe that here, as well.

Before you create your own fact sheet, consult the checklist for or-

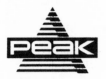

PERFORMANCE CONSULTATION

Dana C. Ackley, Ph.D.
(540) 774-1927

Louis A. Perrott, Ph.D.
(540) 989-8896

FACT SHEET

Peak Performance Consultation helps companies eliminate the psychological barriers to productivity.

- We help employers create work environments that summon exceptional effort from their people, and
- We help executives and supervisors develop skills that can increase productivity in themselves and those who report to them.

Through consultation and training, the firm helps transform companies with "good enough" performance into ones with exceptional or peak performance.

Peak Performance Consultation addresses problems that plague most businesses: conflict management, communications, leadership skills, toxic stress syndrome, the emotional consequences of downsizing, psychological responses to trauma at work, and adapting organizations to new situations. Working with these areas offers business largely untapped ways to multiply productivity.

Peak Performance Consultation differs from other firms in three ways:

- Our training and experience make us experts in change. We know that lasting change can only occur from the inside out. We know why people resist change. We help them recognize and overcome resistance to good change.
- Every project is custom designed. Rather than give predetermined, stock answers, we pay attention to the differences among people and among companies.
- All our work starts with good assessments, which set the foundation for effective solutions.

Today's successful businesses are *learning environments* for their employees. Talented employees want to work where they can develop their skills. Companies that value employee learning keep their best people. Others keep their worst. **Peak Performance Consultation** helps companies find, keep, and develop the best people.

Peak Performance Consultation proprietors Dana C. Ackley, Ph.D., and Louis A. Perrott, Ph.D., are psychologists. Each has over twenty years of experience developing clients' skills. Their scientific training in the laws of human behavior has taught them ways to solve the human problems that come to work with people. Solving these problems is how business will develop productivity and profits in the 21st Century.

3635 Manassas Drive, Suite A • Roanoke, Virginia 24018 • FAX (540) 989-8893

FIGURE 12.2. Fact Sheet for Peak Performance Consultation.

BOX 12.1. Checklist for Organizing Fact Sheet

1. Mission statement *with vision of benefits to the client.*
2. Areas of consultation *with vision of benefits to the client.*
3. Differentiation of the consultant or firm *with vision of benefits to the client*
4. History of firm or consultant(s) *with vision of benefits to the client.*

---

ganizing a fact sheet (see Box 12.1). You may prefer to reorder the elements, but keep uppermost in mind the importance on ending each section with a vision of the benefits that can accrue to the client.

Biographical Sketch

The goal of the biographical sketch is to present you in a way that establishes your expertise and credibility. It should include material relevant to your business consulting, not the material likely to be of interest to consumers of your clinical services. Material of interest to your old professors at graduate school is also to be *excluded.* You will find useful material when you review your history (as outlined in Chapter 9). Remember to write in business friendly language, not professional jargon — jargon creates barriers.

My sketch (see Figure 12.3) was prepared as I was beginning to do business consulting. The one I use today includes additional projects and experiences. However, I wanted you to see what I began with. My experience did not allow me to say that I had been doing business consulting for 20 years. On the other hand, I did not want to write a bio that in effect said: "You would never want to hire me because I have no relevant training or experience." I had to take what I had and make the most of it without being misleading. It took a bit of thought. It required me to review my career with an eye toward seeing how the experiences I had acquired along the way were now relevant to these new endeavors.

Descriptions of Services

Finally, you can develop descriptions of your services. I have included some samples of ours (see Figures 12.4a–12.4c). The goal is to give the company an idea of what you can do *and the benefits to them.* We want to find ways to give them permission to have the problem without feeling "sick."

Design your marketing materials with brevity in mind. While there is a lot I like about our materials, this is one area that can be improved.

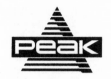

PERFORMANCE CONSULTATION

Dana C. Ackley, Ph.D.
(540) 774-1927

Louis A. Perrott, Ph.D.
(540) 989-8896

DANA C. ACKLEY, Ph.D.

Dr. Ackley works with the wide range of human problems that hinder individuals from working and living to their full ability. He has been a practicing psychologist since 1973. His psychological training lays the foundation for his expertise in helping people and human organizations change.

Dr. Ackley sees people about the problems they have on their jobs and the personal problems they take with them to work. Issues of productivity, performance, leadership, and interpersonal cooperation have occupied a large part of his consultations. In addition, employers have asked him to help their organizations. Such opportunities have included:

- Helping an employer develop systematic ways of working with troubled employees. The result was the first EAP in the Roanoke Valley. It led to significant improvements in productivity and lower medical costs.
- Resolving conflict by improving communication between line supervisors and upper management. The improved atmosphere led to better line supervision and to action plans that solved several accumulated problems. More got done with fewer people.
- Responding rapidly to aid employees exposed to unexpected trauma at work. These interventions prevented serious emotional reactions that often lead to employee resignations, expensive health problems, disability claims, and law suits.
- Assessing candidates for job placement. This results in a better fit between personal skills and job demands. This, in turn, increases productivity and reduces turnover.

Dr. Ackley developed the **Virginia Marketing Project** for the Virginia Academy of Clinical Psychologists. Its goal is to create strategic partnerships between business and psychologists in lowering health care costs and increasing productivity. Executing this program involved, in part, helping to lead a cultural change for this 600+ member organization. This change helped transform a dispirited organization into one of vision and action. The Project has become a national model, and Dr. Ackley has become a national leader in articulating the vast potential of strategic partnerships between business and psychologists.

Leadership and innovation have been prominent in Dr. Ackley's professional life. He was among the first psychologists to establish a successful private practice in the Roanoke Valley, starting in 1977. In 1980 he co-founded The Manassas Group, now the largest group of therapists in the area. He has developed and operated several clinical programs and served

3635 Manassas Drive, Suite A • Roanoke, Virginia 24018 • FAX (540) 989-8893

FIGURE 12.3. Biographical sketch for Dana C. Ackley, Ph.D.

as Director of Psychology for a local hospital. He was a facilitator for the Explore Project during its early years of controversy. Dr. Ackley trained at Hanover College, the Florida State University, and the University of Rochester Medical Center.

Dr. Ackley is in demand as a communicator. Audiences at all levels find his presentations understandable, practical, entertaining, and energizing. His clients include the Practice Directorate of the American Psychological Association, the Independent Practice Division of the American Psychological Association, and the Virginia Psychological Association. His goal in those presentations is for psychologists to better understand how they are uniquely positioned to help business productivity. Local clients have included the Mental Health Association, Roanoke County Schools, Roanoke City Schools, Salem City Schools, Roanoke Memorial Hospital, and Lewis-Gale Psychiatric Center. Local radio, television and newspaper reporters regularly use Dr. Ackley as a resource. He has written several articles for national publications.

FIGURE 12.3. (*cont.*)

Many people experienced in business have told us: "You cannot underestimate the attention span of a CEO." By this they *don't* mean "You shouldn't underestimate it" or "You'd better not underestimate it." They literally mean that any estimate you might make of a CEO's attention span, no matter how short, would not be short enough. Part of this may relate to the personality makeup of people driven enough to become CEOs. Most of it, however, is based not on personality but the realities of their lives. Everybody wants the CEO's attention. Your communications must be concise if you want them to be heard.

This is a serious issue with us because we are such a highly verbal group. Given the choice between expressing a thought briefly or not briefly, not briefly usually gets the nod. This is death in the business world. Many of the subtle distinctions among concepts and the musings that mean so much to us are lost on executives. This is not an issue of intellect. It is an issue of the demands of their world. For their business to be successful, they must make decisions, take care of practical issues, and move along. There is a lot to do, most of it urgent. If we take up a lot of their time with verbosity, they will see to it that we don't get another chance to take up *any* of their time.

6. How Can You Establish Your Credibility?

Credibility is everything. If you establish that you are a credible source of expertise and service, you have done a major portion of gaining the sale. The question, then, is how to gain such credibility.

Our first instincts may be wrong. Under conditions of high performance anxiety, highly educated people typically regress to behavior appropriate to oral exams in graduate school. We become strongly tempted

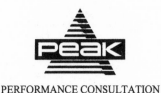

PERFORMANCE CONSULTATION

Dana C. Ackley, Ph.D.
(540) 774-1927

Louis A. Perrott, Ph.D.
(540) 989-8896

WORKPLACE TRAUMA:

CORPORATE RESPONSE PLANS

You don't want to read this brochure. People don't like to think about frightening things that can happen at work - terrible accidents, robberies, disgruntled former employees, random violence. Yet we know that such events occur all too often these days.

By definition, trauma is **frightening AND unexpected.** This leads some people to ignore the possibilities, leaving them without a plan. While we shouldn't dwell on the possible traumas of life, we don't have to hide our heads in the sand either.

Corporations can plan for traumas just as they plan for other possibilities. Employees who witness or survive on-the-job traumas have predictable emotional needs. Meeting those needs within 24 to 48 hours prevents long-term emotional damage.

When emotional reactions to trauma are ignored, many employees, including those whose basic emotional health is sound, can have serious emotional repercussions. High medical costs, periods of disability, and declines in productivity often follow. Many employees leave their jobs altogether, unable to face the reminders of the terror. Angry employees may file law suits.

To be ready for the unexpected, companies today are developing **Trauma Response Plans**. Such plans allow them to act quickly when disaster strikes.

Peak Performance Consultation can help companies prepare and execute **Trauma Response Plans**. We help companies know what needs will exist and how best to handle them. Then, if the time comes, we're there with you to implement them.

3635 Manassas Drive, Suite A • Roanoke, Virginia 24018 • FAX (540) 989-8893

FIGURE 12.4a.

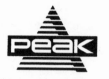

Dana C. Ackley, Ph.D.
(540) 774-1927

Louis A. Perrott, Ph.D.
(540) 989-8896

PERFORMANCE CONSULTATION

DIAGNOSING AND FIXING ORGANIZATIONAL FLAWS

The Problems:

(1) Organizations change.

- What worked for a new organization may not fit one in "mid-life."

- What worked when certain people were present may no longer fit as those people leave and are replaced.

- What was effective under one set of external circumstances may be ineffective as circumstances change.

Organizational flaws can develop unnoticed. While dramatic change is obvious, most change evolves one day at a time. Old responses to new situations or to new people may be increasingly ineffective, reducing productivity and profit. Human nature often leads us to hold onto the familiar, even when it no longer pays.

(2) It is often difficult to know if problems exist because of *organizational issues* or because of the behavior of one or more *people* in the organization. The signs of problems are always in how people act. Are they acting badly because of their own problems, which they inflict on the organization OR are they acting badly because of hidden problems in the organization itself? Fixing the problem relies on knowing the answer to that question. Human nature leads us to personalize problems, i.e., blame somebody rather than look at the organizational level. That can be a costly mistake.

The Solution: "Diagnosing and Fixing Organizational Flaws" is a seminar/consultation program for the management team responsible for organizational effectiveness. The seminar provides conceptual tools the team can use to:

- Distinguish between organizational problems and people problems.

- Understand organizations in a way that improves decision making and problem solving.

FIGURE 12.4b.

The consultation program helps the team to develop and carry out solutions. If a person-centered problem is identified, PPC consultation can help obtain (1) counseling for situations resulting from troubled but valuable employees, or (2) skill-building programs for talented employees with skill deficits for their particular job.

If an organization-centered problem is identified, consultation can help the executive team make needed changes. The PPC role is to focus on the process of change, the center point of our expertise. This allows the executive team to concentrate on the content of the change, the center point of their expertise.

Signs of Problems

How does a company know if a problem exists that requires intervention? We can help you make that decision with a formal assessment. However, you can see a lot for yourself. Consider the following areas (check those that apply):

____ poor morale, such as complaining, whining, an air of chronic tension

____ decreased or poor work quality

____ decreased or poor productivity

____ excessive accidents, absenteeism, disciplinary actions, grievances, disability claims for stress, EEO complaints

____ complaints of fatigue, boredom, decreased motivation, and burnout

____ high turnover, especially when the best people are leaving

____ too many episodes of poor judgement

____ unsatisfied customers

____ high level of unproductive conflict

Signs of Well Being

Look for signs of things going well along with signs of problems (check those that apply):

____ a clear commitment to quality service

____ a sense of urgency in the air, high energy

____ evidence of creativity and innovation - people come up with ideas

____ good people stay

____ high degree of company loyalty

____ satisfied customers

____ an air of trust and communication among all levels

FIGURE 12.4b. *(cont.)*

The Peak Performance Process: The keys to success for this program are the same for success in most endeavors - careful planning, thoughtful execution, and follow-up: (1) We begin with a careful assessment of the company's situation. (2) We use that assessment to tailor the seminar to the needs of the company. (3) We carefully and thoughtfully conduct the seminar. (4) We develop our role in consultation, based on what the seminar and pre-seminar assessment show. (5) We follow-up with the company on the action plans selected.

Investment: This program is always individually tailored. We will be happy to provide a quote based on our discussion of the company's particular situation.

FIGURE 12.4b. *(cont.)*

to show just how much we know and what clever experts we are. But, as your mother told you, no one ever learned anything by talking. Those of us with doctorates get tempted to rely on our title, but the word "Doctor" cuts very little ice in establishing credibility with business. In fact, it can be a problem in two ways. First, it enhances the "shrink" image which makes people defensive. Second, there is a lot of one-upmanship involved in that title. One-upmanship creates barriers, not credibility.

My marketing materials, including my business card, contain "Ph.D." and my biographical sketch discusses my training. However, I do not call myself doctor but rather operate on a first-name basis. I neither hide nor emphasize the word "psychologist." This leaves me free to be flexible in presenting myself. If people want to know a lot about my background, they will ask. If they are more interested in how I might approach their problem, that is what we will discuss. I want to respond to their interests and issues, not my anxiety. My partner likes to use the term "business psychologist," which also has its pluses and minuses.

There are a number of pathways to credibility. Use those that suit you, your experience, your business plan, and your marketing goals. Each of us must create credibility using what is at our own disposal. To illustrate the process, I will share two examples, mine and Saul Gellerman's.

By the time Saul Gellerman had completed his doctorate in clinical psychology, he knew he wanted to be a psychologist within the business community rather than practice therapy. His first job involved doing executive assessments. Before long, he found himself employed by IBM. The IBM time provided him with great experience in functioning within a large corporate culture. When he decided to leave IBM to open his own consulting practice, he wanted to continue working with large corporations.

His way of establishing credibility was to scan the business journals

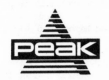

Dana C. Ackley, Ph.D.
(540) 774-1927

Louis A. Perrott, Ph.D.
(540) 989-8896

PERFORMANCE CONSULTATION

THE DOLLARS AND SENSE OF PEAK PERFORMANCE

It's simple, really! Companies that are responsive to the needs of their employees make more money. Research findings are clear about this.

- Companies identified in The 100 Best Companies to Work for in America were found to be twice as profitable as the average Standard & Poor's 500 company.

- Over a 20-year span, progressive companies had higher long-term profitability and financial growth than did those that did not use progressive human resource programs.

- A five-year study by Dennis J. Kravetz found that highly progressive companies had profit margins averaging 5.3% whereas less progressive companies averaged only 3.3%

- Companies using participative management techniques were found to have higher financial strength, more earnings per share, and greater net profits than other companies, as well as less employee turnover, absenteeism, and grievance activity.

Progressive management techniques place **higher demands** on the company's people skills.

Peak Performance Consultation specializes in helping companies bring out the best in their people. Our training and experience helping people change and improve their performances gives us a depth of understanding that helps your company expand its people management skills.

Five additional forces in the workplace demand expanded people skills:

1. Jobs today emphasize Total Quality, teamwork, and attention to customers. These factors require that the hearts, bodies, and minds of employees function optimally.

2. America's "melting pot" is now at work! The traditional workplace is beginning to fill with more females, workers of other races and cultures, and the disabled. Different backgrounds make it harder to communicate, creating more likelihood of conflict and misunderstandings.

3635 Manassas Drive, Suite A • Roanoke, Virginia 24018 • FAX (540) 989-8893

FIGURE 12.4c.

3. The pace of change is quickening. More worker adaptation is demanded, adding to already high job stress. Inadequate adaptation to change leads to physical distress and eventually job burnout. Workers lose motivation as they are stretched beyond their limits. Productivity suffers.

4. The old worker/company contract has been shattered. Companies are no longer able to guarantee lifetime work. In response, employees no longer guarantee unquestioning loyalty. The new employment expectation calls for flexible employee commitments in exchange for personal and professional growth.

5. In the past wide barriers were erected between work and personal life. Personal problems were not expected to intrude on job performance; employers were not supposed to ask about them. Today it is accepted that work and personal life are more integrated, largely because of the changing nature of the workplace.

Each of these changes puts **more demand** on the interpersonal and psychological functioning of company leaders and employees. To maximize productivity, companies must be increasingly knowledgeable

about change,
about **what goes on inside-the-skin of employees,** and
about **interpersonal behavior**.

PEAK PERFORMANCE CONSULTATION SPECIALIZES IN THESE AREAS.

FIGURE 12.4c. (*cont.*)

read by executives in large companies. He learned about the issues of urgent concern to them. He then began submitting articles to those journals, written in their particular style, making it easier for editors to accept them. When the articles were published, he got calls from readers and thereby developed leads to follow up. As a published author who wrote about issues of urgent concern to his target audience, he had established his credibility. Consulting contracts followed.

Saul's method fit his experiences, his personality, and his business plan goals. My approach is based on different resources. I have lived in the Roanoke Valley for 20-odd years and have an established reputation as a competent professional and respected member of my community. It occurred to me that this is a major asset. I decided to make use of that asset via local networking. That approach also fits my business plan, which includes doing most of my work locally.

My primary method of establishing credibility for myself as a business consultant has been to seek out people I already know and talk with them about my new project. Some of these people are potential consulting clients, and others are people who *know* people who may be potential clients. Thus far this strategy has yielded good results as well as some rejections.

SPECIFIC STRATEGIES FOR COMMUNICATING VALUE AND ESTABLISHING CREDIBILITY

Networking

To mount a networking campaign, ask yourself two questions: "Who do I know who is a potential client?" and "Who do I know who knows potential clients?"

When I first asked myself both "who do I know" questions, my responses were "Nobody." So I thought some more. Then came the answer: "*Nobody!*" Then I thought even more and one possibility occurred to me. After the first one came, I managed to eke out one more. Once I had two, it was not hard to get five. As I thought some more and talked to people already on the list, the list began to grow geometrically. My list of networking candidates is now so long that it would take me at least a year to work through it. Having done several projects already, I know that, by the time the next year is up, my portfolio of experience will begin to generate business itself.

So, how to start this brainstorming? Who have you done business with in your community? Did you establish a friendly relationship? Maybe they would be interested in reciprocating. Or maybe they would like to help out a good customer by referring you on to people *they* know. If they allow you to use their name, that is a way of establishing credibility with someone you do not yet know.

Your clinical practice may hold possibilities outside of your therapy clients. In my clinical work, a strong relationship developed with a local school system, one of several in the area. We have done many favors for each other over the years, and many people within the system have referred students and families to my clinical practice. Therefore, I knew that I had credibility with the leaders of this system. The result of my initiating calls to them was a training contract for their assistant principals.

Were you ever an employee in your community? If so, did you work with anyone who might now be a candidate for networking? When I first came to Roanoke, I worked for a private psychiatric hospital. A woman came to work there whom both Lou and I enjoyed working with. Even after leaving the hospital, we kept track of each other. Her children are roughly the same age as mine, so, when we run into each other, we are interested in catching up on family news, etc. I also know her husband, who happens to be a therapist. Several years ago, Lou and I did her a favor related to some community work she was doing, a fascinating experience in and of itself.

Today her job puts her in a position to deal with many business leaders. She is a dynamo and well respected in the community. We took her to lunch to discuss what we are doing. She already believes in our credibility and responded with enthusiasm to our new project. She gave us a list of perhaps 40 local CEOs whom she thought might be receptive. "Use my name." she offered. You cannot buy that kind of credibility.

Review the people with whom you have worked collegially in the past. Where are they now? Are they in a position to offer you business? Are they in a position to offer you credibility by referring you to potential candidates they know?

What about your personal life? Have your nonprofessional activities led you to get acquainted with people who now know you to be a decent human being? That is a beginning in establishing credibility. You are already past the "shrink" image with them. My younger son was interested in joining a number of sports teams during his elementary school years. I volunteered as assistant coach for many of the teams. Fortunately, my severe talent deficiency was overlooked in favor of my ability to offer "sage" psychological input to various coaches. Through these experiences, I met a number of parents, most of whom were grateful that I was assistant coach and they weren't. One man I met is a senior executive in the local office of a major U.S. corporation. When the time came, I called him. Because of our association through our children, he was willing to put me in touch with the decision maker in his organization.

Who have you met through your nonprofessional involvement in the community? Who do you know through your children who recognize that you are a credible human being? Perhaps you have been an assistant coach, or a PTA volunteer, or a church member. This is often how business is done because people prefer to do business with a known quantity. If they know you in these or other ways, and conclude that you have personal integrity, you are already way ahead of unknown competition.

So, who have you met through your personal relationships? Do not ask personal friends for business. Do tell personal friends about what you are doing because they might make a referral.

What about your colleagues? They may be in a position to help. A colleague of mine was asked to participate in a leadership development program for corporate CEOs. For a variety of reasons, the program did not suit him. Because he knew about Peak Performance Consultation, he referred the request to me. Do your colleagues know what you want to do? Who might they refer to you — and who might you refer to them? Find out. Talk about it.

For me, networking fits my requirements and plays to my strengths in communicating value and establishing credibility within what I have defined as my market. Perhaps it will for you too. It has the following advantages:

- It is wonderfully cost-effective, when compared to a major advertising campaign, such as Proctor & Gamble might do to introduce a new product. I don't know about you, but I do not have P & G's financial resources.
- It makes use of some natural experience that professionals have when they have been in a community for even just a few years.
- Because professionals have often done networking to establish their clinical practice, they usually have some experience with it.
- Networking has been extremely helpful in educating me about business issues in my local community. Remember that step 1 in marketing is figuring out what people in your market want.
- People-Consulting in the Workplace is an individualized service. Networking is an individualized approach that fits what you are trying to sell.

Direct Mail

Think again about the material you developed for your "leave-behind." It has additional uses. One is that you can put together a mailing list of target companies. Start sending them a piece from your materials once a month or so. It may function in a way similar to a newsletter. It may begin to build a readership, and people on your list may become familiar with your name. If your material is tasteful and professional, it may leave a good impression. If you happen to strike the right chord at the right time, as Gellerman's journal articles did, you may get a call. By sending diverse materials on a relatively frequent basis, your chances of eventually striking the right chord go up. Not leaving everything to chance, however, you can begin to make follow-up phone calls after sending out a few months' worth of material.

Presentations

Another way to communicate your value is to give presentations. These can be given to the organizations (detailed earlier) that cater to business people. In most organizations, somebody has the problem of finding this month's speaker. Solve his or her problem. However, they will not want you to give a marketing pitch, even though everyone in the room will know that you are marketing. They will want you to speak to something of interest to their members. You can do this in ways that leave your audience interested in your material, interested in you, and with the idea that you have valuable expertise. Bring your leave-behinds to the presentation for people to take home if they wish.

You do have interesting things to say. Be sure you know how to say them in interesting ways. Use language that fits the business world. Use humor, tastefully. Use good audiovisuals. They do not have to be of laser-show quality (although, if you are a technophile, you can learn to do some wonderful things). Do not allow your audiovisual material to be pedantic. Never, never, never read your overheads or slides. Your audience can read. Restate your slide or discuss it but do not read it.

If you get serious about using presentations to attract business, or in using them in your training/consultation work, review *Active Training: A Handbook of Techniques, Designs, Case Examples and Tips,* by Mel Silberman (1990) (see the Appendix). It provides excellent information about how to make presentations to a business audience.

The Media

Another way to communicate your value is through the media. Make a connection with the business editor of your local paper and local business publications. They have to fill a certain number of "column inches" every week. Help them solve that problem. Make an appointment to let them know of your expertise so that they can call on you when they have stories needing such information. Local television and radio programs have similar needs. Read Marcia Yudkin's book (1994) if you decide to go the media route.

SELLING

Let's say that you have now developed a set of services that have potential benefit to business. You have developed a business plan for the delivery of those services. Marketing materials are ready. You have developed and begun to execute your marketing plan. You have delayed as long as you can. Now you must face the issue of going out to sell yourself and your services.

How do marketing and selling relate to each other? Marketing and selling are the same in that both processes involve learning about needs and letting people know that you have answers to those needs. Marketing can be thought of as working with groups. Selling is one on one; it is personal.

The idea of selling raises the anxiety level of many of us to new heights. What follows is designed to reduce your anxiety by: (1) showing you how selling and therapy involve some of the same behaviors; (2) enhancing your selling skills; and (3) providing you with a series of steps that can serve as a desensitization program.

Your Mind-Set

Selling has long been anathema to therapists, among whom the picture of slick, deceptive, sales practices that take advantage of people's weaknesses comes too readily to mind. Such a picture *should* be anathema to us.

In the clinical realm, slick sales practices are particularly dangerous because people usually seek our services during times of psychological vulnerability. Under such circumstances, people are easily misled. When we approach a business, we are unlikely to find that level of vulnerability. Most business organizations have more ego resources than a troubled individual. The potential for you and the company to approach each other on an equal power footing is much higher. In fact, many therapists may feel one-down, which is inconsistent with our more usual experiences. This may be one of the anxiety factors for us.

The mind-set that works well, with both therapy clients and companies, is that you and they each have expertise. The goal is to combine those areas of expertise to solve problems. In addition, each of you has something of value the other wants. Your services have value to companies. Companies have money, which you need to make a living. This mind-set enhances the chance of a good outcome because it is the foundation for a win–win solution. When someone is really in a one-down position, the chances for win–lose become dramatically higher. This is always an inferior outcome no matter who is on the "winning" side.

Getting the Appointment

Before you can sell anything, you have to get an appointment with someone in the company. To set what follows in context, all of my sales calls have been to people I already know or to someone with whom I have a mutual acquaintance. This is consistent with my marketing strategy of networking. Therefore, I cannot provide you with experience-based information on making cold calls.

I am often asked, "How high up in the company should you start?" The easy answer is to start with the company's CEO (chief executive officer, a.k.a. the boss). However, my marketing strategy does not always give me access to the CEO. My approach is to start with the highest person I know, either directly or by referral. That person becomes my company contact.

My strategy for getting appointments comes straight from a sales training seminar that we took from Ronald Lambert of EMME Associates, in Richmond, Virginia (see the Appendix). EMME Associates is a sales training firm. That is all they do. As an experiment, they offered this seminar to volunteers for the Virginia Marketing Project. What a help it was!

The approach Ron taught us has been effective for me whenever I use it to call people I know or people to whom I have been referred. Ron told us that during their training day with regular sales people, the trainers send participants out to the phones to make cold calls for appointments using this approach. Most of the participants came back into the room with appointments.

The purpose of making the phone call is to get an appointment. That is all you want to accomplish. If you get confused on this point, you may talk too much. Then you may never get your appointment, or you may fumble it away. You want to give people enough information so that they can decide whether or not to see you but no more. The more information you give, the more reasons they have to say "no." Further, your call is an intrusion. Business people are more accustomed to intrusions than we are, but it is still an intrusion into an already full day. Therefore, it is polite (and smart) to be as brief as possible.

Anxiety over making these calls is to be expected. Novices like us feel it, and so do well-seasoned sales people. Do not let the anxiety itself become a barrier. After all, you have overcome many other anxiety barriers. One aid is to have a written script in front of you. You may or may not follow it, but you will be more comfortable if you know it is there to fall back on.

My script for the call goes like this: "Hello, John [remember I'm calling someone I know]. This is Dana Ackley [followed by a brief pleasantry]. The reason I'm calling is that I am offering some new services designed to remove psychological barriers to employee productivity. I have some ideas that I think might be of interest to you. I'd like 20 to 30 minutes of your time to discuss them with you. Would Wednesday afternoon, at 2:00, work for you?" If you get an agreement, repeat the time, day of the week, date, and place. (You will be amazed at how often one of you will get this wrong.) "Great! Then I'll see you Wednesday at 2:00 at your office."

The steps in this call are:

- Identifying yourself
- Establishing a reason for calling that is designed to appeal to the person called
- Asking for a *minimal* commitment
- Providing structure about when to meet

This script is based on already knowing the individual. If you do not know the person, the call can be modified: "Hello, Mr. Smith. This is Dana Ackley. I believe you know Joyce Jones, who suggested that I call you. I am a business psychologist who is offering services to remove the psychological barriers. . . . "

Sometimes you will get an appointment, and sometimes you will encounter resistance. You need not be fearful of resistance because all of your professional training and experience have helped prepare you to handle it. Ron suggests the LAER method for dealing with resistance: Listen, Acknowledge, Explore, and Respond.

- *Listen* to understand why they are resisting. Perhaps there is something you can do to overcome the resistance. You might hear: "I am really crunched for time right now."
- *Acknowledge* to show that you understand: "I can understand that this is a busy time for you. My schedule has been a bit crazy, too." This sends the message that you not only understand his time problem but that you identify with it and that you are not messing around either.
- *Explore* to achieve an alternative: "Would another time be better?" Maybe three weeks later the crunch will not be so severe.
- *Respond* to explain or clarify. Suppose the objection was not time but something like: "I don't think we have those kinds of problems here." This person may be responding to the pathology image associated with therapists. He is giving you a chance to respond to his concern before he decides about your request. Your response might be: "Maybe not, but you will be surprised at the number of things we can do to help even well-run companies improve their worker productivity. Keeping everyone pulling in the same direction is a full time job. If we got together we could spend a few minutes talking about how companies that are doing well can do even better."

Rejection

Sometimes, you won't get an appointment. Isn't it interesting how much anxiety anticipated rejection can create? Let's consider what Albert Ellis might say. He would tell us that it is not the rejection we fear but rather it is our own interpretation of its meaning. While we cannot control whether we get rejected, we *can* control our interpretation of it. One reality-based interpretation is that rejections will occur no matter how well we perform on the phone.

Sometimes, companies just are not ready for us when we want them to be ready. If we get nothing but rejections, we might decide that we are not making the calls correctly, but that is a fixable condition. Some unrealistic interpretations are that the services offered have no value, or that companies have no need, or that we ourselves are without value. The truth is that not even the experts get an appointment every time. They just keep trying.

The Sales Visit

Homework

You need to do some homework on the company. Find out what business they are in, who the key executives are, and whether there are any recent news stories that will give you useful information. Check out the library for reference materials, such as the *Million Dollar Directory*.

The Appointment Itself

Now you are off to see a potential client. You are wearing business professional clothing. What can you expect? It may surprise you to learn that selling and therapy have three things in common: (1) listening is fundamental; (2) the focus of the encounter is on the client, not you; and (3) you must have faith in the value of your services, or you should not be offering them.

Listening Is Fundamental

When I began making sales calls, I relied heavily on our list of services. I used it as a "prop" in opening conversations. This encouraged giving content intensive information about the various services. (When clinicians become nervous, we usually become content intensive.) This turned out not to be useful. Potential clients would listen attentively, ask polite questions and say "We'll get back to you." When I shifted my focus from me and my list to them and their needs and interests, I was more successful. In other words, I found ways to hear what the company needed rather than pushing what I wanted to sell.

The following procedure seems to work well: Begin a meeting with the obligatory small talk. This is good business etiquette and has the advantage of allowing each of you to size up the other. Not good at small talk you say? Neither am I. That does not make it impossible. Thinking of the individual as a human being, rather than just a possible client, opens up your mind to ways of relating before getting down to business.

Next, talk briefly about your services. I try to do this in about 4 minutes, literally. I plan to find a way to finish with something like "We deal with people problems in the workplace." The response is often some version of "Boy, do we have those here!" If you do not get some version of that response, you are unlikely to sell services to that company.

If you do get that kind of response, it is time to shut up, listen, and let the people tell their story. The stories are usually quite interesting, so the listening is not hard. Ask questions. The act of active listening, so rare in business life, begins to create a bond between you and potential clients. As people are talking, you will often find that you begin to have ideas about the kinds of interventions that might be useful. Your excitement about the possibilities probably will become evident as you pursue the topics. If your excitement is genuine, it can only add to the client's interest in you.

Perhaps you can see how this is similar to seeing new therapy clients. We usually do not know what kind of therapy services we will offer to the clients as we move toward the chairs to sit down. We have to listen to their story first. As they talk, however, ideas begin to emerge. It is the same with People-Consulting in the Workplace.

Sometimes, as the listening goes forward, ideas will not come. Do not let that worry you. Turn it to your advantage. You can say something like: "That sounds like a tough problem. I think we can do something really interesting with it. Let me give it some thought and get back to you with some ideas. How about next Thursday for lunch?" An advantage of this response is that you have agreed that it is a tough problem and made it clear it will have individual attention. There will be no canned response. In addition, you have bought some time and created a reason to get back together.

It Isn't About You

Neither therapy nor selling is about you. Both are about the client or potential client. Neither is a measure of your performance or competence. This shift in focus will reduce your anxiety level immensely and open you to genuine listening and relating.

Think about the advice you might give to someone during sex therapy. We know that if participants in a sexual experience are focused on measuring their performance, rather than enjoying the experience and considering the other person, anxiety ruins both the experience and the performance. Likewise, when we do therapy, or make a business call, it is not about us, either. It is about the client. That is where our focus should be. As long as you keep your focus on the potential client, it will be easy for you to access your interest, energy, and expertise. Clients will often respond to this genuine interest with pleasure.

Our role in selling People-Consulting in the Workplace services is to provide companies an opportunity they may never have had before. Their needs might be intense, but if they do not know about our services or how to access them, the services will remain out of their reach. As we talk with them, we can help employers conceptualize what will be useful in their particular situation.

Provide Value

Just as you would not provide bogus therapy services, do not sell services to business that you do not have faith in. You may encounter situations in which you are asked to do things that you know are not right or will not work. Don't. First, it is not worth the lost sleep. Second, it will discourage the company from buying appropriate services because they already know your integrity level.

> I was 5 minutes away from winning an agreement for a lucrative consulting contract. We were hammering out the last few details when a sudden flash of insight made me realize that we were going down the wrong path. There was no way that what the leaders of this company were asking for would provide the value they sought. Their lack of psychological expertise made the service look good to them. It was my job to notice the problem, which I did just before it might have been too late. I called a halt to the negotiations, telling them that our plan was not going to work: "Let me think about how else we could do this and call you next week." They agreed. The following week we came to an agreement that worked well for them, for their employees, and for me.

The Two Basic Methods of Selling

Ron Lambert taught us that there are two basic approaches to sales: (1) "I have the best widget" and (2) "What widget do you want?" He encouraged us to use the second approach.

First, from a technical sales point of view, option 1 is a tougher sell. If the company is already buying widgets from someone else, you must convince them that your widgets are superior. To do this, you must disrupt an ongoing relationship, which is not easy. Basically you have to convince them they have been making a mistake.

Second, from a professional ethics point of view, it also creates problems. We do not want to be in the position of saying that our services are superior to everyone else's. We want to talk about our value without running others down. We do not want to imply that we are the only ones who know the secret ways to productivity.

Option 2 emphasizes listening. To figure out which widget is wanted or needed, you must listen carefully to what is being said. This is your strong suit, anyway—why not use it? You tailor your services to the unique needs and wishes of your therapy clients. Do the same in business.

Tip. If you can help your contact in the company look good in the eyes of the CEO, the chances of your getting a contract are high. Obviously if your services are likely to make your contact look bad to the CEO, you will get nowhere. Your contact cannot afford to put himself in jeopardy. If he sponsors you to the company, he is betting some part of his credibility on your performance.

The easiest service to sell is one that answers the problem that keeps the CEO up at night. Everyone in the company is oriented around what worries the CEO. Ask what that problem is. If you are not meeting with the CEO, ask your contact what the CEO's mission is for his or her tenure. What are the issues that he or she feels are most urgent. Answers to these questions can yield critical information.

Do not expect to sell a contract at the first meeting. It almost never happens. The rule of thumb in sales is that it takes five contacts to make a sale. Not every contact has to be a meeting. A phone call is a contact; a letter is a contact; and so forth.

You will get rejected sometimes. Remember to be careful about how you interpret that outcome.

Desensitization

When I began getting ready to make sales calls, my anxiety level went through the roof. I fabricated reasons why I could not make a call "just now." That *increased* my anxiety. Not only was I allowing my fear to build, but I was also standing in the way of my own progress. I had to find a way to break this destructive cycle. What I came up with was a plan to take action in manageable steps. In this way I could lessen my anxiety, both by desensitizing myself to it and by countering it with action. Perhaps it will be useful to you:

- *Step 1.* Role play some calls with a friend. This will give you a chance to practice getting the words organized and to get some feedback. You may even want to videotape your practice calls so you can review them.
- *Step 2.* Set up a few appointments with some of your network candidates. The goal of these meetings is not to sell anything. It is to seek advice and feedback on your plans from some actual business people. This is what Lou and I had in mind when we had that lunch meeting with the husband of my real estate broker, who ran his own company. You will get a chance to present your ideas in a near sales call setting and get some friendly reactions. You will feel less performance anxiety.
- *Step 3.* Make a few calls on some real candidates with whom you see little likelihood of getting a sale. What this will do is give you a chance to present yourself in a real sales situation without the pressure of feeling that you "must succeed." You should not ex-

pect to. One experience we had was to call on someone who in her old job had been a referral source. She now works for one of the local governments. I knew we would get a warm reception from her, but that the chances of actually getting business were small. Again, performance anxiety was minimized.

- *Step 4.* Now, in earnest, begin to call on good possibilities. By now you have some background and experience, which will help you manage your anxiety.

The Proposal

During your initial sales call, you want to be looking for an opportunity for another contact. (Remember, it takes five.) Offering to prepare a proposal often fits this bill nicely.

Remember that the chances of selling something in your first meeting are small. This is not surprising because you are still in the building stage of your relationship. The function of the "five contact rule of selling" is that people need to establish some kind of minimal trust with you before they are willing to purchase the kinds of services you are proposing. Having several contacts allows each of you to get to know the other well enough to know if you want to take the relationship to the next stage.

The similarities between establishing a business relationship and establishing a therapy relationship are worth noting. Therapy clients do not trust us instantly, either. They and we find ways to spend time with each other until the bond is strong enough to do the more difficult work.

Imagine now that you are nearing the end of an initial sales call that feels promising. The rapport feels good. A reasonable amount of candor has developed. You have the beginnings of an idea about the problems the company is facing. You may be beginning to formulate an intervention, even if it is only a means of assessment. What now?

Now you want to create a reason for another meeting. If your contact is the decision maker, you will want your next meeting to be with this same person. If the decision maker wants to involve other key players in the next meeting, so much the better. If your contact cannot make the decision about hiring you, work toward connecting with the decision maker.

As the initial meeting is winding down, paraphrase the problem you are hearing until you get agreement that you have heard it accurately. Be sure you know what steps the company has taken to solve the problem so far. Float some trial balloons to see if your initial ideas might have promise. This will help assure that your written proposal will not be a plan that the company would reject out of hand, and you along with it. If you get some interested response to your trial balloons, say something like: "This is an interesting problem. It seems we might be on the track of something that may help. I would like to put these ideas in the form of a written proposal. I will mail that proposal by (name a date). Then I would like to meet with you (and the decision maker, if you can swing it) a few days later (name a date and time) to talk about it." Secure an agreement to this plan.

If you do not have ideas or if you want to do some research before offering your initial thoughts, that is fine. In that case, you can say: "This is an intriguing problem. I can see why it has been hard to solve. I would like to give it some thought and get back to you with a written proposal. I will get something to you by (name a date) and then why don't we meet to go over it a few days later (name a date and time)." This response acknowledges the difficulty the problem presents to the company. Before you actually send something in writing, however, you may want to call your contact to review the broad outlines of your proposal, again to avoid proposing something that the company is already unwilling to consider.

Proposals need to be written concisely, and they need to use business language, not our professional jargon. Do not use research citations. Business people tend to view academic types as impractical. The business mentality is to be practical and action oriented. Business does value research but tends to be much less rigid about what research looks like than our graduate school professors were.

The outline I have found useful for proposals is:

- Statement of the problem
- History of the problem
- Proposed approach
- Rationale
- Rough time frame
- Financial terms of the contract

This is the outline I have in my head. I do not necessarily actually use these titles. You can modify the outline depending on the situation. I offer it just to give you some structure as you do your first first few proposals.

What follows is a sample proposal based on a real situation, but, as with all other illustrations in the book, the facts have been changed to protect individual and company privacy. The problem outlined is common to many companies, that of supervisors or managers who are technically skilled but not trained in interpersonal skills required in effective management. The project was eventually accomplished, though not exactly as outlined in this proposal. The proposal served as structure for our ongoing discussion. That discussion allowed me to learn more about what would be helpful. Jointly, the leadership of the company and I modified our plans until we were all satisfied enough to proceed.

Date

Names of addressee
Company name
Address

Dear X:

It was good to meet with you the other day and hear about the recent progress made by your company. The personnel processes you have been putting in place over the past several years clearly have been paying off in terms of production per employee and long-range leadership development. As you noted, these are ongoing processes, not issues that respond to an easy fix.

We discussed how Peak Performance might help you take the next step. You expressed concerns about how supervisors deal with the interpersonal aspects of supervision. Their skills in understanding the technical aspects of their jobs are superior, but they tend to have problems knowing how to deal with line employees. Then, when things get hot, they get their superior to handle the problem. Their superior already has many duties. The company needs the supervisors to take more responsibility for their own personal leadership of employees.

The specific goals you set to be accomplished next are to improve the interpersonal skills of your supervisors and help their assistants learn these skills so that they will be ready to step into supervisory positions in the future.

This could be done in a 4-step process:

1. Assessment. In line with the Peak Performance process, step 1 is an assessment of the needs of the supervisors and assistants. The assessment began with our discussion the other day. Next I would interview a few of the people to be trained from each level to get their input and to have a more direct feeling for their skill level. Time required: 4 hours.

2. Building motivation. I would then consult with you and the trainees' superior on the development of strategies to enhance participants' motivation to learn additional supervisory skills, given that we can anticipate some reluctance. Time required: 1–2 hours.

3. Initial training. A 2- to 4-hour workshop will be given to the group. The actual length and specific content will be determined by the assessment process and the motivational strategies we develop. The goals are to present useful information and to initiate a positive relationship between participants and trainer. It may work best to split the group in two, offering the program twice. Hopefully, this would allow you to maintain production, and the smaller size might help the group atmosphere. We can decide later whether it is best to do the training on-site or at a nearby facility. Time required: 4–8 hours.

4. Ongoing Training. Growth in supervisory skills will only happen if three conditions are met: participants are motivated to learn, believe they can learn, and the learning occurs within a relationship with a trainer that is both comfortable and challenging. These goals can be approached in two ways.

One is a group consultation format, which can work well if the initial group training experience really clicks. This method would have participants meet as a group to look at actual supervisory problems they have had to face. This allows us to use the expertise of the participants, as well as the expertise of the trainer, as they work to help each other with common problems.

The alternative approach is one of individual coaching. In this approach, I would be available 2 hours per week. Interested supervisors could sign up for time slots to consult on problems they are facing.

We can decide which format to use after step 3 has been completed. I suggest we run the program initially for three months. Then we can evaluate progress and decide whether to continue, modify, or discontinue. Total time required, regardless of format: 26 hours.

INVESTMENT: $7,800 to $8,800, depending upon the time required.

I will call you in a few days to set up a meeting in which we can review this proposal.

Sincerely,

Dana C. Ackley, Ph.D.

The Project

We eventually settled on a training program on conflict management, a good place to start in terms of interpersonal skills. This program can be presented in a nonshaming way because conflict is ubiquitous. During the assessment phase, supervisors discussed with good candor the real-life conflicts that existed in their company. They agreed that everyone can improve conflict management skills.

The training was conducted in two phases. The first phase involved group based didactic and mildly experiential work. The second phase involved individual meetings with each participant to discuss any work-based interpersonal issues the participant wanted to discuss. The initial group sessions were tough, but, as our relationships developed, we found ways to work together. Once we were "over the hump," the participants did a great job of working with the material. During our individual meetings, participants looked at issues that were of pressing concern to them in dealing with their supervisees.

The content of the training sessions led to discussions of conflicts within this particular company. With the understanding I developed as a result of these discussions I was able to propose related consultation projects. The first of these was to help the company with some issues around management structure, including some team-building work. This experience helped all of us realize that the original training goal could not be fully achieved until some attention was paid to company culture. Company leadership became greatly interested in tearing down old barriers among work groups that were now blocking optimum productivity. New patterns of communication began to develop, which supported the supervisors in their work of improving their own interpersonal skills.

My consultation experience with this company was extremely satisfying. The people involved were interested in making a real contribution to their company and to one another. Knowing the people involved as individuals is "proof positive" that some of our long-standing impressions of "how business people are" have been misimpressions indeed. What I have found are human beings who work with human issues as well as they can with the tools at their disposal. As their tools improve, so do their results.

SUMMARY

In this chapter we have discussed the nitty-gritty issues of how to market and sell consultation services to business. My goal was to give you enough tools to get started. Some of this material is probably new information for you. However, some of it may be more familiar than you would have guessed. That is part of the point. What you already know is much more applicable to People-Consulting in the Workplace than you might have thought. You already have many of the skills you need. They just require a little adaptation, imagination, and action.

Afterword

Well, there you have it. You have the basic intellectual and practical tools you need to begin to market and sell your services without depending upon insurance and managed care companies. My guess is that most of the ideas make sense to you. What are the barriers now to your getting started?

I will take a chance and guess that one of your barriers will be forcing yourself from a thinking mode to an action mode. We tend to be *idea* people. We are often not people of action. Yet, ideas alone will not save you. You must start. You must act. The secret is momentum. The smallest act can be the beginning of your managed care free practice.

We ask our seminar participants to write to us to report their initial steps. Some people begin by buying a Rolodex or calling a bank about accepting credit cards. Some throw out managed care contracts. Others make lists of people to call, find a buddy, create new marketing materials, develop new services, rewrite office policies, or sign up for a training program. They go on from there.

The transition of your practice from third-party dependent to third-party free will take time. No, I am not talking about transition, although that will take time too. I mean you must devote time to making it happen. At a minimum, devote 1 hour per week to this process. If you work a 40-hour week, this 1 hour represents 2.5% of your workweek. Make the investment.

If possible, find a buddy to work with. It is hard to move against conventional wisdom by yourself. If people tell you what you are doing is impossible, listen selectively. They may help you to recognize barriers you will need to overcome. But do not get hypnotized by negativity. Choose to hang out with people who think the way you do. Encourage each other.

Your biggest obstacles at this point are likely to come from within yourself. Like our clients, we can get frozen by fear of change. Talking with your friends can help you identify emotional obstacles and get past them. You might even want to form a support group of therapists in your area who have decided to establish private pay practices. The support I experience from therapists from all over the country who are working in these directions is a powerful factor in sustaining my emotional energy. Remember that, if you have successful competitors, they are making it more normal for people to use the kinds of services you are trying to provide. That kind of competition creates more business to be shared.

Finally, write to me. Let me know how it's working. Let me know what you are discovering. I will pass it along to others through the newsletter that has grown out of our seminars. During these rough times, we need to hold each other's hands.

Appendix:
Annotated Resources

In developing the model for a managed care free practice, a number of sources of information and training have been of great help.

1. Robert H. Rosen, Ph.D., with Lisa Berger. (1991). *The healthy company*. New York: Tarcher/Perigee.

   Rosen is a clinical psychologist who has been applying psychological concepts to the business world for the past decade. His book, though written for the business audience, outlines for therapists the countless ways that we can apply what we already know in a work setting. He also presents data about the cost effectiveness of such undertakings. This book can be used as a resource for therapists moving into People-Consulting in the Workplace.

2. David B. Walters, Ph.D., and Edith C. Lawrence, Ph.D. (1993). *Competence, courage, and change: An approach to family therapy*. New York: Norton.

   This excellent book on family therapy was written by two experienced clinical psychologists. Its special relevance to us is that it concisely outlines many aspects of the Problem-Solving and Skill-Building model. Therapists interested in developing effective clinical services that bypass the damaging impact of preoccupation with pathology will find articulate support here.

3. Lyn Payer. (1992). *Disease-mongers: How doctors, drug companies, and insurers are making you feel sick*. New York: Wiley.

   Payer is a medical reporter who presents a well-researched examination of the medical model applied not just to mental health but across the entire spectrum of disorders. The dangers of applying the model both in the psychological realm and in more traditional areas of health are cogently presented.

4. J. R. O'Neil. (1993). *The paradox of success: A book of renewal for leaders.* New York: Tarcher/Putnam.

   O'Neil is President of the California School of Professional Psychology. In addition, he has a long-standing consulting practice to business leaders. In his book, O'Neil presents Jungian concepts to business leaders in a startlingly understandable way. This book can provide you:

   • A better understanding of some of the psychological issues faced by successful business leaders.
   • A resource that you can recommend to your business consultees.
   • An understanding of why therapists have been so reluctant to give up the medical model even after it no longer helped us.

5. Stephen R. Covey. (1989). *The 7 habits of highly effective people: Powerful lessons in personal change.* New York: Fireside.

   Covey was educated in business (M.B.A. from Harvard) and teaches management. Yet, he has learned a great deal about our area of expertise—change. This runaway best-seller can help therapists to understand how some of our concepts look to business people now and how we might adapt them better to business use in the future.

6. Ken Pelletier. (1992). *Mind as healer; mind as slayer.* New York: Dell Publishing.

   Pelletier is a research and consulting psychologist who has done much of the cutting-edge work in health promotion, especially in developing such programs within the business community. This book is probably the only stress management book you need. Pelletier's workshops on health promotion are also excellent preparation for taking this information to the business community.

7. David M. Noer. (1993). *Healing the wound.* San Francisco: Jossey-Bass.

   Noer is a business consultant who has learned a great deal about how emotional well being affects productivity. In this book, he turns his attention to the emotional devastation most downsizings generate, which most companies downsizing fail to consider. As a direct result of this failure, such companies almost always lose (lots of) money in the process. Those companies that do attend to the emotional elements in downsizing do much better. Although Noer did not review the psychological research literature, I have. His comments and insights are strongly supported.

8. J. Keith Murninghan. (1992). *Bargaining games: A new approach to strategic thinking in negotiations.* New York: William Morrow.

   This is a fun book to read. It contains many exercises that you can adapt to fit into conflict management training workshops. It will also give you some tools to use in negotiating contracts for yourself.

9. James M. Kouzes and Barry Z. Posner. (1987). *The leadership challenge: How to get extraordinary things done in organizations*. San Francisco: Jossey-Bass.

   This book and its accompanying workbooks will help you design leadership training activities. It helps readers understand the basics of leadership, describing leadership as a set of skills that many people can learn. Business desperately needs help in learning how to train its managers to lead. Supplement this volume with the excellent review article on psychological research relevant to leadership in the June 1994 issue of *American Psychologist* (Hogan, Curphy, & Hogan, 1994). It will demonstrate to you that we really do know a lot that can be useful in this area.

10. Mel Silberman. (1992). *20 active training programs*. San Diego: Pfeiffer & Co.

    This resource provides ready-to-go outlines for 20 training programs you may want to offer to business. I found some of more interest than others. Handouts and overheads that you can reproduce are included. They allow you a way of getting started immediately. Alternatively, they provide a beginning outline you can modify for yourself. In my experience, companies like it when you offer them customized training programs rather than something canned. These outlines, however, give you a beginning point.

11. Mel Silberman. (1990). *Active training: A handbook of techniques, designs, case examples and tips*. New York: Lexington Books.

    This is a companion book to the preceding source. It provides excellent advice and information on how to do training. Many of you will already know much of this material, while others may not. Veterans will find the chapters a useful checklist for details as they are putting together a program. New trainers will find this a useful primer, enabling them to avoid otherwise predictable mistakes.

12. *Pfeiffer & Company* publishes a wide variety of training materials. Some of the sources cited here can be obtained through them. To receive their catalogue, call 800-274-4434.

13. *University Associates,* a company associated with Pfeiffer & Company, provides some excellent seminars. These are largely oriented to trainers in the business community. They provide some basic information that has been quite helpful, enabling me to feel less like I was on foreign soil when I went to business. "Organizational Development" and "Facilitating Organizational Change" were exceptionally well run and provided good fundamental information. Their telephone number is 520-322-6700, fax 520-322-6789.

14. *Frank Taylor* is the marketing consultant I hired for the Virginia Marketing Project. His insights and faith in our profession were integral to the development of People-Consulting in the Workplace. Prior to beginning his own

consulting practice, he had 25 years of experience as a senior executive with Blue Cross. Thus, he knew how therapists really got into trouble with managed care and helped us gain that perspective. Therapists who are serious about developing a competitive place in their market would benefit from his counsel: 9702 Gayton Road, Box 300, Richmond, VA, 23233. Telephone: 804-741-7704.

15. Jay Conrad Levinson. (1993). *Guerrilla marketing: Secrets for making big profits from your small business.* Boston: Houghton Mifflin.

This is a basic marketing book oriented toward small businesses, not IBM. It is well written and easy to follow. It will have some ideas unsuited to professional practice. However, many of his thoughts are likely to be useful to you and may lead you to fresh ideas of your own.

16. Jay Conrad Levinson and Seth Godin. (1994). *The guerrilla marketing handbook.* Boston: Houghton Mifflin.

This is a companion piece to *Guerrilla Marketing.* It provides much additional information, some in the form of sources of various services that may be useful.

17. *Ronald Lambert* is the president of *EMME Associates,* a sales training company in Richmond, Virginia. He provided the sales course several of us therapists took that was mentioned in Chapter 12. It was extremely helpful. Telephone: 804-330-4115.

18. *Creative Dimensions in Management* is the group that does culture change for corporations by doing therapy with the leading executives. They also hold workshops for therapists to learn how this is accomplished. Address: 1100 East Hector Street, Suite 200, Conshohocken, PA 19428. Telephone: 610-825-8350.

19. *Ivan Miller, Ph.D.,* has established one of the first "marketing guilds" for therapists interested in building practices outside managed care. A guild is a good mechanism that solo practitioners and small group practices may wish to employ to pool marketing resources while maintaining their autonomy. Ivan has established one model of how to do such a guild and is interested in sharing this model with others. Address: 350 Broadway Street, Suite 210, Boulder, CO 80303. Telephone: 303-444-1036.

20. *The National Coalition of Mental Health Professionals and Consumers, Inc.* is a national organization with a growing number of state affiliates. As the name suggests, members include both professionals and consumers. Its goal is to respond in a number of ways to the dangers created by managed care. Led by Karen Shore, Ph.D., the goals of the Coalition are to educate professionals and the public regarding the serious problems with managed care, to

work for legislative reforms to help regulate the managed care industry, and to support the development of more humane forms of third-party reimbursement.

Those who have read this book know that I do not believe that our future, or the future of our clients, lies with third-party reimbursement. However, we are in a time of change, a period during which a variety of responses are evolving to the managed care problem. As organizations and movements mature, differentiation of ideas and opinions naturally occurs. However, what the Coalition and I *do* share is a serious concern about the impact managed care is having on the services available to people. No other organization has, to my knowledge, done more to educate the public about the problems involved with managed care than has the National Coalition. They will gratefully accept your dues and your involvement. Address: P.O. Box 438, Commack, NY 11725-0438. Telephone: 516-424-5232

References

Ackley, D. C. (1993). Employee health insurance benefits: A comparison of managed care with traditional mental health care: Costs and results. *Independent Practitioner, 13*(1), 33–40.

Ackley, D. C. (1995). Beyond managed care: Creating alternatives while keeping the faith. *Family Therapy Networker, 19,* 71–75.

American Psychological Association Practice Directorate. (1995). *Violence in the workplace.* Washington, DC: Author.

Antonuccio, D. O., Danton, W. G., & DeNelsky, G. Y. (1995). Psychotherapy versus medication for depression: Challenging the conventional wisdom with data. *Professional Psychology: Research and Practice, 26*(6), 574–585.

Associated Press. (1995, June 6). New study shows link between profit and employees. *Roanoke Times and World News, 36,* p. 341.

Austad, C. S., & Hoyt, M. F. (1991). The managed care movement and the future of psychotherapy. *Psychotherapy, 29,* 109–118.

Bak, J. S., Weiner, R. H., & Jackson, L. J. (1991). Managed mental health care: Should independent private practitioners capitulate or mobilize? *Texas Psychologist, 43,* 23–37.

Barkley, R. A. (1990). *Attention-deficit hyperactivity disorder: A handbook for diagnosis and treatment.* New York: Guilford Press.

Barkley, R. A. (1995). *Taking charge of ADHD: The complete, authoritative guide for parents.* New York: Guilford Press.

Barlow, D. (1991). *The treatment of anxiety and panic disorders.* Conference sponsored by the Mid-Atlantic Educational Institute, Absecon, NJ.

Berkman, L. F., Leo-Summers, L., & Horowitz, R. I. (1992). Emotional support and survival after myocardial infarction. *Annals of Internal Medicine, 117,* 1003–1009.

Borus, J. F., Olendzki, M.C., Kessler, L., Buens, B. J., Brandt, U. C., Broverman, C. A., & Henderson, P. R. (1985). The offset effect of mental health treatment on ambulatory medical care utilization and changes. *Archives of General Psychiatry, 42,* 573–580.

Broadhead, W. E., Blazer, D. G., George, L. K., & Chiu, K. T. (1990). Depression, disability days, and days lost from work in a prospective epidemiological survey. *Journal of the American Medical Association, 264*(19), 2524–2528.

Brody, D. S. (1980). Physician recognition of behavioral, psychological and social aspects of medical care. *Archives of Internal Medicine, 140,* 1286–1289.

Chopra, D. (1993). *Ageless body, timeless mind.* New York: Crown.

Chua-Eoan, H. G. (1992, Fall). Life in 999: A grim struggle. *Time* [Special Issue], p. 18.

Coopers and Lybrand. (1995). *Positioning psychology in the marketplace: Trends and strategies.* In R. E. Bachman (Chair), Symposium conducted at the American Psychological Association State Leadership Training Conference, Washington, DC.

Corrigan, P. W. (1995). Wanted: Champions of psychiatric rehabilitation. *American Psychologist, 50*(7), 514–521.

Covey, S. R. (1989). *The 7 habits of highly effective people: Powerful lessons in personal change.* New York: Fireside.

Cummings, N. A., Dorken, H., Pallak, M.S. (1990). *The impact of psychological intervention on healthcare utilization.* California: Biodyne Institute.

Cummings, N. A., & Follette, W. T. (1968). Psychiatric services and medical utilization in a prepaid health plan setting, Part II. *Medical Care, 6,* 31–41.

Depression a big cost to business. (1993). *Roanoke Times, 156*(34), p. 6.

Did you know? (1995, Summer). *Advance, 5.*

Dobson, K. S. (1989). A meta-analysis of the efficacy of cognitive therapy for depression. *Journal of Consulting and Clinical Psychology, 57,* 414–419.

Elkind, D. (1981). *The hurried child.* Reading, MA: Addison Wesley.

Ellis, A. (1987). The impossibility of achieving consistently good mental health. *American Psychologist, 42*(4), 364–375.

Fiedler, J. L., & Wight, J. B. (1989). *The medical cost offset effect and public health policy: Mental health industry in transition.* New York: Praeger.

Freeny, M. (1995, September/October). Do the walls have ears? *Family Therapy Networker, 5*(19), 37–43, 65.

Goleman, D. (1995). *Emotional intelligence.* New York: Bantam.

Gonik, U. L. et al. (1981). Cost-effectiveness of behavioral medicine procedures in the treatment of stress-related disorders. *American Journal of Clinical Biofeedback, 4*(1), 16–24.

Gorman, C. (1996, May 6). Who's looking at your files? *Time,* pp. 60–62.

Gravelle, J. (1993, July 4). Conflicts among workers found to hurt bottom line. *Roanoke Times, 34*(4), p. F3.

Gray, J. (1993). *Men are from Mars, women are from Venus: A practical guide for improving communication and getting what you want in your relationship.* New York: HarperCollins.

Hammer, M., & Champy, J. (1993). *Reengineering the corporation: A manifesto for business revolution.* New York: Harper Business.

Hankin, J. R., Kessler, L. G., Goldberg, I. D., Steinwachs, D. M., & Starfield, B. H. (1983). A longitudinal study of offset in the use of nonpsychiatric services following specialized mental health care. *Medical Care, 21,* 1099–1110.

Harrison, P. A., & Hoffman, N. G. (1989). *CATOR report: Adult inpatient completers one year later.* St. Paul, MN: Ramsey Clinic.

Hayashida, M., Alterman, A. I., McLellan, A. T., O'Brien, C. P., Purtill, J. J., Volpicelli, J. R., Raphelson, A. H., & Hall, C. P. (1989). Comparative effectiveness of inpatient and outpatient detoxification of patients with mild-to-moderate alcohol withdrawal syndrome. *Journal of Studies on Alcohol, 52*(6), 517–540.

Heinssen, R. K., Levendusky, P. G., & Hunter, R. H. (1995). Client as colleague: Therapeutic contracting with the seriously mentally ill. *American Psychologist, 50*(7), 522–532.

Herron, W. G., Javier, R. A., Primavera, L. H., & Schultz, C. L. (1994). The cost of psychotherapy. *Professional Psychology: Research and Practice, 25,* 106–110.

Hogan, R., Curphy, G. J., & Hogan, J. (1994). What we know about leadership: Effectiveness and personality. *American Psychologist, 49*(6), 493–504.

Holder, H., Longabaugh, R., Miller, W. R., & Rubonis, A. V. (1991). The cost effectiveness of treatment of alcoholism: A first approximation. *Journal of Studies on Alcohol, 52*(6), 517–540.

Howard, K. I., Kopta, S. M., Krause, M. S., & Orlinsky, D. E. (1986), The dose–effect relationship in psychotherapy. *American Psychologist, 41*(2), 159–164.

Hunter, R. H. (1995). Benefits of competency-based treatment programs. *American Psychologist, 50*(7), 509–513.

Jansen, M. (1986). Emotional disorders in the labour force: Prevalence, costs, prevention and rehabilitation. *International Labour Review, 125*(5) 605–615.

Jones, K. (Ed.). (1979). Report of a conference on the impact of alcohol, drug abuse, and mental health treatment on medical care utilization [Supplement]. *Medical Care, 17,* 1–82.

Kamlet, J. S., (1990). *Depression in the workplace: Issues and answers.* Baltimore: National Institute of Mental Health: Depression Awareness, Recognition, and Treatment.

Kazdin, A. E. (1993). Psychotherapy for children and adolescents: Current progress and future research directions. *American Psychologist, 48,* 644–657.

Kessler, L. G., Steinwachs, D. M., & Hankin, J. R. (1982). Episodes of psychiatric care and medical utilization. *Medical Care, 20,* 1209–1221.

Kessler, L. G., Cleary, P. G., & Burke J. D. (1985). Psychiatric disorders in primary care. *Archives of General Psychiatry, 42,* 583–587.

Kiecolt-Glaser, J. K., Malarkey, W. B., Chee, M. A., Newton, T., Cacioppo, J. T., Mao, H. Y., & Glaser, R. (1993). Negative behavior during marital conflict is associated with immuological down-regulation. *Psychosomatic Medicine, 55,* 395–409.

Kiesler, D. J., & Wagner, C. C. (1992). *The modal number of sessions for brief psychotherapy: One managed care program's guideline and the research evidence.* A report to the Virginia Academy of Clinical Psychologists. Unpublished manuscript, Virginia Commonwealth University.

Koocher, G. P. (1994). Preventive intervention following a child's death. *Psychotherapy, 31*(3), 377–382.

Kouzes, J. M., & Posner, B. Z. (1987). *The leadership challenge: How to get extraordinary things done in organizations.* San Francisco: Jossey-Bass.

Kovacs, A., & Albee, G. (1975). Comments on "insurance reimbursement." *American Psychologist, 30*(12), 1156–1164.

Kronson, M. E. (1991, April). Substance abuse coverage provided by employer medical plans. *Monthly Labor Review,* 3–10.

Kuttner, R. (1991). Sick joke: The failings of managed care. *New Republic, 205,* 20–22.

Layton, M. (1995, November/December). Mastering mindfulness. *Family Therapy Networker, 19*(6), 28–30, 57.

Levinson, J. C. (1993). *Guerrilla marketing: Secrets for making big profits from your small business.* Boston: Houghton Mifflin.

Levinson, J. C., & Godin, S. (1994). *The guerrilla marketing handbook.* Boston: Houghton Mifflin.

Lewin, M. H. (1978). *Establishing & maintaining a successful professional practice.* Rochester, NY: Professional Development Institute.

Lowman, R. (1991). Mental health claims experience: Analysis and benefit redesign. *Professional Psychology: Research and Practice, 22*(1), 36–44.

Maddi, S. R., & Kobasa, S. C. (1984). *The hardy executive: Health under stress.* Chicago: Dorsey Professional Books/Dow Jones-Irwin.

Manning, W. G., Wells, K. B., Duan, N., Newhouse, J. P., & Ware, J. E. (1984). Cost sharing and the use of ambulatory mental health services. *American Psychologist, 39*(10), 1077–1089.

Marshall, J. (1993, November 3). Downsizing isn't the cure-all people are looking for. *Richmond Times-Dispatch, 93,*(310).

Massad, P. M., West, A. N., & Friedman, M. J. (1990). Relationship between utilization of mental health and medical services in a VA hospital. *American Journal of Psychiatry, 147,* 465–469.

McDonnell Douglas Corporation and Alexander Consulting Group. (1990). *Employee Assistance Program Financial Offset Study: 1985–1989.*

McClellan, A. T., Luborsky, L., O'Brien, C. P., Woody, G. E., & Druley, K. A. (1982). Is treatment for substance abuse effective? *Journal of the American Medical Association, 247*(10), 1423–1428.

McNeilly, C. L., & Howard, K. I. (1991). The effects of psychotherapy: A reevaluation based on dosage. *Psychotherapy Research, 1*(1), 74–78.

Meichenbaum, D. (1989, May 12–13). *Cognitive behavior modification: Effective interventions with adults, children and adolescents.* Symposium conducted at the Conference on Cognitive Behavior Modification, Washington, DC.

Mental health: Does therapy help? (1995, November). *Consumer Reports,* pp. 734–739.

Michelson, L. K., & Marchione, K. (1991). Behavioral, cognitive, and pharmacological treatments of panic disorder with agrophobia: A critique and synthesis. *Journal of Consulting and Clinical Psychiatry, 59*(1), 100–114.

Moldawsky, S. (1990). Is solo practice really dead? *American Psychologist, 45,* 544–546.

Moyers, B. (1993). *Healing and the mind.* New York: Bantam, Doubleday, Dell.

Mumford, E., Schlesinger, H. J., Glass, G. L., Patrick, C., & Cuerdon, T. (1984). A new look at evidence about reduced cost of medical utilization following mental health treatment. *American Journal of Psychiatry, 141,* 1145–1158.

Murnighan, J. K. (1992). *Bargaining games: A new approach to strategic thinking in negotiations*. New York: William Morrow.

Noer, D. M. (1993). *Healing the wound*. San Francisco: Jossey-Bass.

O'Neil, J. R. (1993). *The paradox of success: A book of renewal for leaders*. New York: Tarcher/Putnam.

Orleans, C. T., George, J. K., Houpt, J. L., & Brudie, H. K. (1985). How primary care physicians treat psychiatric disorders: A national survey of family practitioners. *American Journal of Psychiatry, 142,* 52–57.

Payer, L. (1992). *Disease-mongers: How doctors, drug companies, and insurers are making you feel sick*. New York: Wiley.

Pelletier, K. R. (1991). A review and analysis of the health and cost-effective outcome studies of comprehensive health promotion and disease prevention programs. *American Journal of Health Promotion, 5*(4), 311–315.

Pelletier, K. R. (1992). *Mind as healer; Mind as slayer*. New York: Dell.

Pelletier, K. R. (1993, August 16–20). *Practical strategies for health promotion*. New York: Albert Einstein College of Medicine.

Prodigy News Service. (1995, December 6). What insurers are saying about you. Kiplinger's.

Psychotherapy Finances. (1995, January). Survey report, *21*(1), p. 1.

Psychotherapy Finances. (1995, July). Professional notes, *21*(7), p. 12.

Psychotherapy Finances. (1995, August). Practice issues: He doesn't like managed care—so he stays out of it, *21*(8), p. 1.

Quinn, J. B. (1996, May 6). Tuition increases haven't cut applications to pricey colleges. *The Roanoke Times, 36*(310).

Reuters News Service. (1983, October 18). *Report: More than 2 million workers attacked on job*.

Rice, D. R., Kelman, S., Miller, L. S., & Dunmeyer, S. (1990). *The economic costs of alcohol and drug abuse and mental illness: 1985*. Report submitted to the Office of Financing and Coverage Policy of the Alchohol, Drug Abuse, and Mental Health Administration, U.S. Department of Health and Human Services. San Francisco: Institute for Health and Aging, University of California.

Robinson, L. A., Berman, J. S., & Neimeyer, R. A. (1990). Psychotherapy for the treatment of depression: A comprehensive review of controlled outcomes research. *Psychological Bulletin, 108,* 30–49.

Rosen, R., with Berger, L. (1991). *The healthy company*. New York: Tarcher/Perigee.

Rosenberg, J. (1995, June 18). CEO counselor sees field change with the times. *Roanoke Times, 34* (168), p. F4.

Schlesinger, H. J., Mumford, E., & Gene, V. (1983). Mental health treatment and medical care utilization in a fee-for-service system: Outpatient mental health treatment following the onset of a chronic illness. *American Journal of Public Health, 73,* 422–429.

Seitz, V. A. (1992). *Your executive image: The art of self-packaging for men and women*. Holbrook, MA: Bob Adams.

Seligman, M. E. P. (1990). *Learned optimism*. New York: Pocket Books.

Sharfstein, S. S., Muszynski, S., & Arnett, G. M. (1984). Dispelling myths about mental health benefits. *Business and Health, 1884,* 7–11.

Sheehan, D., Ballenger, J., & Jacobsen, G. (1980). Treatment of endogenous anxiety with phobic, hysterical and hypochondriacal symptoms. *Archives of General Psychiatry, 37,* 51–59.

Silberman, M. (1990). *Active training: A handbook of techniques, designs, case examples and tips,* New York: Lexington Books.

Silberman, M. (1992). *20 active training programs.* San Diego: Pfeiffer & Company.

Smolowe, J. (1996, April 15). A healthy merger? *Time, 147*(6), 77–78.

Spotlight: Managing stress in the workplace. (1991, March). *Prevention Report, U.S. Public Health Service,* p. 7.

Steenbarger, B. N. (1994). Duration and outcome in psychotherapy: An integrative review. *Professsional Psychology: Research and Practice, 25*(2), 111–119.

Steinbrueck, S. M., Maxwell, S. E., & Howard, G. S. (1983). A meta-analysis of psychotherapy and drug therapy in the treatment of unipolar depression with adults. *Journal of Consulting and Clinical Psychology, 51,* 856–863.

Stewart, D. (1993). *Creating the teachable moment: An innovative approach to teaching and learning.* Blue Ridge Summit, PA: TAB Books.

Taube, C. A., Kessler, L., & Feuerberg, M. (1984, June). Utilization and expenditures for ambulatory mental health care during 1980. *National medical care utilization and expenditure survey data* (Report No. 5). Washington, DC: U.S. GPO, National Center for Health Statistics, Public Health Services.

Taylor, F. (1994). *Competitive edge market study report.* Winchester, VA: Virginia Academy of Clinical Psychologists.

Vaccaro, V. A. (1991). *Depression: Corporate experience and innovations.* Washington, DC: Washington Business Group on Health.

VandenBos, G. (1992). [Personal communication re: Health Service and Research Administration quarterly reports.]

Walker, C. K. (1991, September). Stressed to kill. *Business and Health,* 42.

Walters, D. B., & Lawrence, E. C. (1993). *Competence, courage, and change: An approach to family therapy.* New York: Norton.

Ware, J. E., Manning, W. G., & Duan, S. (1984). Health status and the use of outpatient mental health services. *American Psychologist, 39,* 1090–1100.

Weiner, B. (1993). On sin versus sickness: A theory of perceived responsibility and social motivation. *American Psychologist, 48*(9), 957–965.

Wells, K. B., Stewart, A., & Hayes, R. D. (1989). The functioning and well-being of depressed patients. *JAMA, 262,* 914–919.

Wylie, M. S. (1992). Toeing the bottom line. *Family Therapy Networker, 16,* 30–39, 74–75.

Yudkin, M. (1994). *Six steps to free publicity.* New York: Plume/Penguin.

Index